Gary W. Hartz, PhD
D. Michael Splain, LCSW

Psychosocial Intervention in Long-Term Care
An Advanced Guide

Pre-publication
REVIEWS,
COMMENTARIES,
EVALUATIONS . . .

"**I**n Chapter 5, the authors give the reader useful interventions that will help them communicate with long-term care residents who are diagnosed with Alzheimer-type dementia. Offered in this chapter are ways of achieving empathy and a genuine relationship with this most difficult population. Personnel who work in long-term care will learn to understand the very old resident who cannot see or hear, or has lost his/her family, recent memory, mobility, and a sense of usefulness. Staff will learn that these residents often retreat to the past in order to avoid a painful present reality.

They never prepared for old age. Hartz and Splain recognize that a pure cognitive approach is not always helpful and can cause frustration for staff members. When personnel achieve empathy and understand the reasons behind the disoriented person's behavior, frustration lessens, communication becomes genuine, and burnout is significantly reduced. Personnel report more job satisfaction and staff turnover decreases."

Naomi Feil, MSW
Executive Director,
The Validation Therapy
Training Institute, Inc.

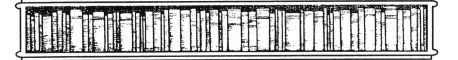

"**P**sychosocial Intervention in Long-Term Care provides social service practitioners with a comprehensive overview of psychosocial assessment and treatment in long-term care. Social service workers will be able to more clearly define their role, and become more integral to the treatment process in long-term care. From the history of nursing home regulations to efforts to reduce psychotropic medication, this book provides new insights for social service practitioners."

Peter A. Lichtenberg, PhD
Associate Professor of Physical Medicine and Rehabilitation, Wayne State University, Detriot, MI

"**F**inally, a definitive guide on psychosocial intervention specifically for long-term care. Hartz and Splain have created an easy-to-read reference and 'how to' in one volume.

I believe that Psychosocial Intervention in Long-Term Care will become the standard required reading for all who deal with the 'whole person' in the long-term care setting. A real achievement, an A+."

Edward G. McMahon, PhD
Vice President of Education, Regency Health Services, Inc., Tustin, CA

"**T**he authors face the reality of long-term care and tell us how to use that reality for the residents' benefit. This book is thorough, well-researched, and practical. It tells us how to do different things in helpful and humane ways. The information in this book is helpful for all long-term care employees no matter their level of experience. It is concrete and clear and the explanations and directions are easy to follow. The authors are advocates for good resident care while teaching long-term care employees how to find satisfaction and effectiveness in their work."

Marylou Hughes, LCSW, DPA
Psychotherapist and Nursing Home Consultant, Ft. Pierce, FL

More pre-publication
REVIEWS, COMMENTARIES, EVALUATIONS . . .

"**P**sychosocial Intervention in Long-Term Care is primarily written for social workers and nurses in long-term care (LTC), but it is a book for anyone in the LTC field. The authors explain issues and techniques with simple, straightforward language and technical expertise. It is an ideal orientation for anyone interested in the psychosocial aspects of LTC. It contains a wealth of practical information and numerous case illustrations for primary LTC providers. It is a solid, technical resource for social workers, nurses, and LTC administrators. Psychologists new to providing mental health services in LTC will find it a one-source handbook. It is probably a book so useful that it should not only sit on a professional's bookshelf, but should be placed right alongside the *PDR* for ready reference by all staff dealing with residents in LTC facilities."

Michael Gilewski, PhD
Clinical Psychologist,
Rehabilitation,
Cedars-Sinai Medical Center,
Los Angeles, CA

The Haworth Press, Inc.

Psychosocial Intervention in Long-Term Care
An Advanced Guide

Psychosocial Intervention in Long-Term Care
An Advanced Guide

Gary W. Hartz, PhD
D. Michael Splain, LCSW

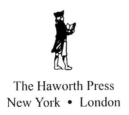

The Haworth Press
New York • London

The Haworth Press, Inc., 10 Alice Street, Binghamton, NY 13904-1580

Cover design by Becky J. Salsgiver.

Original painting by Gretchen McGarigle.

Library of Congress Cataloging-in-Publication Data

Hartz, Gary W.
    Psychosocial intervention in long-term care : an advanced guide / Gary W. Hartz, D. Michael Splain.
       p.   cm.
    Includes bibliographical references and index.
    ISBN 0-7890-0189-6 (alk. paper).
    1. Nursing home patients–Mental health. 2. Geriatric psychiatry. I. Splain, D. Michael. II. Title.
RC451.4.N87H37 1997
362.1'6–dc21
                             96-48819
                               CIP

We dedicate this book to the nursing assistants of long-term care, whose energy, love, and compassion bring light to our residents.

ABOUT THE AUTHORS

Gary W Hartz, PhD, serves as consulting psychologist to seven LTC facilities as part of his San Jose-based private practice. He is also a staff psychologist at the Veterans Affairs Palo Alto Health Care System. Author or co-author of eleven professional articles, his specialties are psychological assessment and behavioral intervention. He is a member of Psychologists in Long-Term Care, the American Society on Aging, the American Psychological Association, the California Psychological Association, and the Santa Clara County Psychological Association.

D. Michael Splain, LCSW, serves as a social services consultant to over sixty LTC facilities in Northern California. He has worked as a social worker in Salt Lake City (he set up the first residential treatment program for adolescents in Utah), a director of a methadone program, and a forensic social worker at the Santa Cruz County jail. Mr. Splain has been working in LTC since the early 1980s; one of his clinical specialties is hypnotherapy, which he integrates into his LTC practice. He is a member of the National Association of Social Workers.

CONTENTS

Preface

Working in long-term care (LTC) has never been more challenging. Residents admitted to nursing homes are older and more disabled than in the past, compounding the psychosocial problems that staff must face. At the same time, pressures are mounting to cut costs aggressively in both the Medicare and Medicaid programs. The combination of these forces means that in the future, staff will have to do more with less. In particular, LTC facilities will likely have fewer staff members to deal with an increased number of psychosocial and behavioral problems.

The future might not be so grim if these pressures were counterbalanced by an increased availability of mental health consultants who were paid by Medicare and Medicaid. However, we believe that in the near future, changes in Medicare and Medicaid reimbursement will make it less likely that nursing home patients will receive services from mental health professionals. The burden of assessing these patients will fall mainly on the shoulders of the social services and nursing staff, who may lack adequate training in the assessment and treatment of psychosocial and behavioral problems.

Specifically, more and more seniors are signing over their Medicare benefits to managed care companies. LTC patients under a managed care plan often do not receive mental health evaluations and treatment from professionals because most managed care companies do not authorize them. The reason for this is that the companies usually have a financial incentive to limit the number of services provided to each patient. Consequently, the LTC staff and physicians are left to do the assessment and design interventions by themselves. This book provides one means of training staff to do this.

This book is designed for social workers, nurses, and other professionals who know some basics of psychosocial assessment and intervention in LTC. Through experience, they have discovered how difficult some of the problems are, and they are now ready to take the next step in their training. This book is thus an "advanced guide," as well as a very practical, hands-on approach to common psychosocial problems.

Because we intend to provide advanced training, we do not address some of the most basic aspects of social services in LTC. These include issues such as resident rights, case management, the resident council, and family support groups. Hopefully, readers of this book understand these basic areas, and are ready to focus on the more complex issues of assessment, intervention, and documentation of psychosocial problems.

While we address the special needs of residents who speak foreign languages, we do not provide an overview of racial and ethnic differences among residents and their families. Here in California, we work with staff and residents from a myriad of backgrounds, and we recognize that these differences can create barriers to communication and care. However, entire books have been written on this issue. Space did not allow for the kind of discussion that would do justice to its complexity.

We have tried to write a book that is helpful to both nonmedical professionals, such as social workers, and medical preofessionals, such as nurses. When it comes to assessing and intervening with psychosocial problems, there is a great deal of overlap in the responsibilities of the medical and nonmedical disciplines. In addition, our biopsychosocial model of assessment and intervention emphasizes the importance of a medical perspective, as well as a psychological and social one.

We should make a clarification regarding the case histories that we describe. We distinguish between "Case Studies" and "Case Illustrations." Most of the cases that we describe are Case Studies, in which all of the material is factual. By contrast, Case Illustrations are fictional cases in which we have created a typical presenting problem and typical interventions that we have successfully used with similar residents.

In order to avoid sex bias in our language, we have tried to use feminine and masculine pronouns equally throughout the book. We have not used "he or she" or "his or her," because they sometimes make sentences too lengthy and awkward.

Organizationally, the book is divided into four main sections. After a brief historical perspective in Chapter 1, the following three chapters concern the assessment of psychosocial and behavioral problems. We describe residents' psychosocial needs and the biopsychosocial model in Chapter 2. In Chapter 3, we discuss mental health evaluations, the Mental Status Examination, and the nature of cognitive impairment and depression. In Chapter 4, we teach the administration and interpretation of the Geriatric Depression Scale and Mini-Mental State Exam. The next four chapters focus upon intervention. In Chapter 5, we provide an overview of counseling techniques; in Chapter 6, we discuss behavioral assessment and intervention; in Chapter 7, we summarize interventions for specific behavioral problems; and in Chapter 8, we discuss the side effects and uses of psychiatric medications. The next two chapters focus upon administrative and legal issues. Chapter 9 explains the Resident Assessment Instrument and highlights key survey issues. Chapter 10 discusses various legal and ethical issues that arise in LTC, and the procedures that are used to address them. Finally, in Chapter 11 we address staff's psychosocial well-being and how they can prevent themselves from burning out.

Acknowledgments

The authors wish to express gratitude to the following staff members of the Veterans Affairs Palo Alto Health Care System who provided helpful and enlightening comments on our chapters: to Steve Lovett, PhD, and Bill Lynch, PhD, for their reviews of Chapter 3 (Assessment of Mental Disorders); to Margaret Florsheim, PhD, for her review of Chapter 4 (GDS and MMSE); to Suzanne Ogland-Hand, PhD, of the Knoxville, Iowa Veterans Adminstration Medical Center, for her review of Chapter 5 (Behavioral Assessment); to Helen Ostruske, LCSW, for her review of Chapter 6 (Psychotherapy); to Jon Rose, PhD, and Dolores Gallagher-Thompson, PhD, for their reviews of Chapter 7 (Psychosocial Interventions); to Bill Faustman, PhD, and James Hawkins, MD, for their reviews of Chapter 8 (Psychiatric Medication); and to Laurie Ackerman, LCSW, for her review of Chapter 11.

We also express appreciation to Barbara Morrey and Ginger Kane, MSW, social services designees, for their reviews of Chapter 4 and trial use of the two instruments. Also appreciated is the review of Chapter 10 by Sidney Chapman, a private professional conservator for Lifespan. We acknowledge helpful insights about possible future trends in LTC from Ed McMahon, PhD; Bill Nicholson; and Yvette Osterhaus.

Great thanks go out to our mentors and advisors: Mack Gift, PhD; Joseph Pendry, LCSW; Randy Parker, LCSW; Brian Small; and the many social workers who work so hard to meet the psychosocial needs of residents that we discuss in this book.

Special appreciation is extended to Clifford Bennett, PhD, for his pioneering work in the field of psychosocial intervention in LTC during the late 1970s. His book has served as an inspiration for our work in this field.

Finally, we express great appreciation to our spouses, Sue Ritter-Splain, MFCC, and Teri Wiss, MA, OTR, for their help and support during this project. Sue edited drafts of several chapters, put them on a word processor, and provided feedback about our chapters. Teri, an Occupational Therapist, provided articles from the OT literature and made helpful comments on four chapters.

Chapter 1

The Past, Present, and Future of Psychosocial Services in Long-Term Care

We keep them alive until 65, then we bury them at 75.

–Jack LaLanne

The demand for long-term care (LTC) has never been greater. Approximately 1.5 million people, or 5 percent of the population over 65 years of age, currently live in LTC facilities (German et al., 1992). Twenty to 50 percent of those over age 65 will eventually spend some time in a nursing home (German et al., 1992). Future demand may be even greater, because the elderly are living longer and their proportion in the population continues to grow.

Given these trends, what is the future of psychosocial services in LTC? In this chapter, we hope to provide a glimpse of the future, but to understand that, we have to study the past. Thus, we start with a look at how nursing homes began and the legislation that affected them over the past five decades. We then summarize the standards for psychosocial services that were common before OBRA 87, as compared with those that are currently required. We finish with a few cautious predictions about the future of psychosocial services in LTC.

A HISTORICAL PERSPECTIVE

During the eighteenth and early nineteenth centuries, the chronically ill were treated in buildings known as poorhouses, pest houses, workhouses, and city and town infirmaries (Bennett, 1980). These served as prototypes for present-day nursing homes, and a few have survived as modern-day hospitals. For example, Pennsylvania Hospital in Philadelphia was founded in 1751 and Bellevue Hospital in New York was founded in 1816. Both were originally established to serve the elderly, disabled, and chronically ill (Bennett,1980).

Passage of the Social Security Act of 1935 marked the beginning of nursing homes as we know them today. This act constituted the first time that the Federal Government assumed a caregiving role for the elderly. Under this act, Congress funded a federal and state public assistance program called Old Age Assistance (OAA), which provided income to needy people over age 65. As a result, "large numbers of aged who were ill or blind left state and county institutions to claim OAA and to reside in boarding homes," which "became nursing homes" (Davis, 1994, p. 2). These were more like "rest homes" or present-day residential care homes. They often had large front porches, attractive gardens, and a capacity of no more than 20 to 30 beds (Bennett, 1980). They were often operated by registered nurses who "were compassionate individuals who wanted to give disabled people more personal care than hospitals delivered" (Bennett, 1980, p. 18).

In 1950, the Social Security Act was amended to create licensing programs for nursing homes which were administered by individual states. This amendment "gave official status to nursing homes" (Davis, 1994, p. 2), and thus spurred the creation of more LTC institutions. Further efforts to support LTC culminated in the Hill-Burton Act of 1954 and a 1956 amendment to the Social Security Act, both of which increased funding for LTC facilities. Consequently, the number of nursing homes mushroomed. Mirroring this trend was OAA's dramatic increase in spending: from $35.9 million in 1950 to $280.3 million in 1960 (Institute of Medicine, 1986).

As part of President Lyndon Johnson's "Great Society" legislation, Medicare and Medicaid were born in 1965. This legislation was the first to set standards of participation which were prerequisites for state and federal funding, and were enforced by the Department of Health, Education, and Welfare (HEW). These standards were derived largely from the regulations of the Joint Commission on Accreditation of Health Care Organizations (JCAHO).

Consequently, they reflected the prevailing medical model and a hospital-oriented system of care (Morford, 1988). Critics charged that these medically oriented regulations emphasized physical safety and sound medical treatment to the exclusion of quality-of-life issues.

From 1969 to 1973, these standards and the LTC industry as a whole were scrutinized by Senator Frank Moss' Senate Committee on Aging. After this long process, a number of reports were published which underscored the problems in LTC facilities. One of the reports provided the following perspective:

> This [nursing home] industry, which has grown very rapidly in just a few decades–and most markedly since 1965, when Medicare and Medicaid were enacted–could now take one of three courses: It could continue to grow as it has in the past, spurred on by sheer need, but marred by scandal, negativism, and murkiness about its fundamental mission. It could be mandated to transform itself from a predominantly proprietary industry into a nonprofit system, or into one which takes on the attributes of a quasi-public utility. Or it could–with the help of Government and the general public–move to overcome present difficulties, to improve standards of performance, and to fit itself more successfully into a comprehensive health care system, in which institutionalization is kept to essential minimum. (Subcommittee on Long-Term Care, 1974)

We underscore this last point about the institutional quality of nursing homes, which is our main concern in the next chapter.

During this time, President Nixon proposed an eight-point plan to improve nursing home regulations. Several of these points were as follows: (1) to centralize Medicare and Medicaid activities; (2) to expand HEW's enforcement activities; (3) to increase funding for training state surveyors; (4) to provide field funding for state nursing home inspection programs; and (5) to decertify substandard facilities. Once it was enacted by legislation, however, this plan was criticized as weak and too general. HEW, on the other hand, defended the regulations as providing performance standards that were flexible enough for evaluating facilities.

In 1974 and thereafter, the Office of Nursing Home Affairs (ONHA) evaluated these revisions and the quality of nursing home care. Its efforts led to the development of an evaluation instrument called "Patient Appraisal and Care Evaluation" (PACE), but this proved too cumbersome as a method of home survey.

In the late 1970s, President Carter initiated his own reform measure, "Operation Common Sense." This spurred both HEW and the Health Care and Finance Administration (HCFA) to revise the survey process for skilled nursing facilities. While the nursing home industry criticized this revision for its extensive review and paperwork requirements, HCFA still published it in 1980. These regulations were the first to use outcome measurements as an index of the quality of care. Specifically, these regulations did the following: (1) consolidated all resident care planning requirements into one condition; (2) required a resident care management system using an interdisciplinary team for assessment and treatment planning; (3) de-emphasized the medical model by reducing requirements for the attending physician; (4) elevated residents' rights to the status of a condition of participation; and (5) combined the Skilled Nursing Facility (SNF) and Intermediate Care Facility (ICF) regulations into a single set called the Code of Federal Regulations (CFR).

However, during the deregulatory atmosphere of the Reagan presidency, these standards were rescinded, which returned us to the 1974 standards. The Health Care and Finance Administration (HCFA) then attempted to streamline the survey and enforcement process by adding new elements of flexibility. They also proposed allowing states to accept private accreditation by the Joint Commission (JCAHO) as sufficient for participating in Medicare and Medicaid. These efforts were met with outrage from certain advocacy groups, who perceived them as an effort to reduce protection for the frail elderly.

HCFA then took two important steps. First, it developed a new protocol called Patient Care and Services (PACS), which used direct patient assessments and outcome-oriented indications of care. The PACS was based on the Patient Appraisal and Care Evaluation (PACE) and was developed through a series of demonstration projects. Second, in 1983, HCFA funded an Institute of Medicine (IOM) study of nursing home regulation. This study culminated in a 1986 report from the Committee on Nursing Home Regulation, which was called "Improving the Quality of Care in Nursing Homes." The committee concluded that residents received "shockingly deficient" care and made recommendations regarding residents' rights, quality of care, staffing, surveys and certification (Coleman, 1991).

The importance of this study was that it provided a national consensus on the changes that were necessary in LTC, and carried with it the considerable prestige and influence of the Institute of Medicine (IOM) (Morford, 1988). HCFA attempted to implement IOM's recommendations by formulating new requirements for participation in Medicare and Medicaid and new enforcement procedures. At the same time, Congress was working to pass nursing home legislation that would implement the IOM recommendations, which brings us to OBRA 87.

Omnibus Budget Reconciliation Act (OBRA)

On December 21, 1987, Congress passed the Omnibus Budget Reconciliation Act (OBRA), Subtitle C, The Nursing Home Reform Act. Passed as Public Law 100-203, the bill amended Medicare and Medicaid statutes in the following LTC areas: quality of life, scope of required services, interdisciplinary assessment, activities, training standards for nurse's aides, physician supervision and clinical records, resident rights, and required social services. Nursing facilities were required to meet specific standards in these areas in order to qualify for Medicare or Medicaid reimbursement. The law also eliminated the distinction between skilled nursing and intermediate-care facilities.

Under OBRA, the Medicaid reimbursement rates were increased to account for the additional cost of meeting these higher standards. However, as more and more regulations have been added since 1987, frustration has mounted among LTC staff, because reimbursement increases have not compensated them for the mounting burden of paperwork.

Psychosocial Services Before and After OBRA

Prior to OBRA, the role of psychosocial services in LTC was loosely defined. Given that nursing homes were viewed largely in terms of health care and medical services, psychosocial issues took a back seat to medical ones. Psychosocial services consisted primarily of attending to concrete personal needs, such as supplying residents with clothing, eyeglasses, and transportation. They also included supportive counseling conducted by nurses, activities directors, chaplains, and community agencies. In fact, there often was no social services designee, and it was the activities director who often had to perform basic social services. Fortunately, OBRA clearly defined the position of social services designee.

Similarly, California's Title 22, which predated OBRA, had little to say about social services, relative to other disciplines. It briefly described a "social work service unit," but this was listed under "optional services." Consequently, few facilities created such a unit. Even more striking is that social services were not even mentioned in the Required Services section of theTitle. Surveyors were left with a highly subjective, loosely interpreted standard for evaluating social services. This standard usually boiled down to the meeting of residents' concrete needs and the completion of initial assessments, discharge planning, and quarterly reports. However, there were states outside of California that recognized the importance of social services and thus required much more of that department.

HCFA's current (1995) requirements for social services are quite specific, as can be seen in the excerpt shown in Table 1.1. More specific criteria for fulfilling these requirements are listed in HCFA's Guidance to Surveyors. An excerpt of these criteria appear in Appendix B at the end of the book, where we discuss their practical implications for surveys.

These guidelines marked the first time that the traditional designee role merged with the contemporary bachelor's and master's level social worker. OBRA made it very clear that social services in LTC were no longer confined to "finding eyeglasses" and "calling families for clothes."

The recently published Minimum Data Set 2.0 (MDS 2.0) extends this emphasis upon treating the whole person. The MDS 2.0 elevated psychosocial aspects of the resident's care to a status equal to that of medical concerns. The importance of psychosocial needs is also underscored by the extensive psychosocial assessments required by the Resident Assessment Inventory (RAI) and the Resident Assessment Protocol (RAP), which we discuss in Chapter 9.

TABLE 1.1. HCFA's 1995 Requirements for Social Services

(a) 483.15 (g) (1): The facility must provide medically related social ser-vices to attain or maintain the highest practicable physical, mental, and psychosocial well-being of each resident.

(b) 483.15 (g) (2): A facility with more than 120 beds must employ a quali-fied social worker on a full-time basis.

(c) 483.15 (g) (4): A qualified social worker is an individual with—

   (i) A bachelor's degree in social work or bachelor's degree in a human services field including but not limited to sociology, special educa-tion, rehabilitation counseling, and psychology; and

   (ii) One year of supervised social work experience in a health care setting working directly with individuals.

(d) 483.20 The facility must conduct initially and periodically a comprehen-sive, accurate, standardized, reproducible assessment of each resi-dent's functional capacity.

   – 483.20 (b) (2) (vii): [This assessment must include] mental and psycho-social status.

   – 483.20 (b) (4) (iv): Assessments must be conducted promptly after a significant change in the resident's physical or mental condition.

Note: Excerpted from "Guidance to Surveyors" (HCFA, 1995).

What Our Survey Has Taught Us

What have we learned about psychosocial services from this brief survey of the history of LTC and psychosocial services? First, there is always tension between two extremes: overregulation and deregulation. The political pendulum swings between these, and the amount and type of documentation required of LTC settings swings with it. Nursing home staff resent bureaucratic burdens that take time away from patient care, yet without these requirements, some institutions might neglect patients. This tension is one that we must learn to live with.

Second, while the idea of treating the whole person is an old one, the practice is a recent development. Well-rounded psychosocial services became a requirement only when OBRA 87 took effect; thus, the field has just emerged from infancy. This makes the field of LTC psychosocial services an exciting one because many creative ideas have yet to be born.

THE FUTURE OF PSYCHOSOCIAL SERVICES IN LONG-TERM CARE

Predicting the future is always risky, but if we look closely at present trends and future demographics, we get some good clues. We mentioned the future demographics at the beginning of this chapter. Concerning present trends in the health care arena, they are as follows: (1) the minimizing of hospital stays by rapidly moving patients to lower-cost LTC facilities or to skilled nursing units within the hospital; (2) the use of a wider range of assisted-living and home-based health care options before placing someone in LTC; (3) the proposed cuts in Medicaid and Medicare funding; (4) the development of capitated, or managed-care, reimbursement plans for medical services covered by Medicare and Medicaid; and (5) increasing numbers of seniors who have LTC insurance policies. These trends, combined with projected demographics, lead us to the conclusions below.

First, *a greater proportion of LTC Residents will be extremely disabled.* The proportion of severely disabled residents in LTC appears to have risen over the last decade, and this is likely to continue. One reason for this trend has been the concomitant expansion of alternatives to LTC, such as home care and assisted living. Assisted-living centers will continue to expand the nursing services that they offer, so that only the most severely disabled must be transferred to nursing homes. Another reason is that many hospitals have short-term nursing home units for their previously hospitalized patients. Many of these patients have acute or postoperative problems that do not demand long-term placement.

Second, *less disabled residents will be discharged faster.* For residents who can recover functional abilities after a medical crisis, managed care companies will be quite motivated to discharge them from LTC as quickly as possible. This may lead to shorter stays and a higher turnover of residents.

Third, as we discussed in the Preface, *social services and nursing staff will have to do psychosocial assessments and intervention themselves, with occasional help from consultants.* Managed care companies are not likely to authorize mental health consultants' evaluations and treatment, and LTC facilities will probably only pay for such in severe cases.

Fourth, under managed care plans, *residents will receive reduced amounts of occupational, speech, or physical therapy.* This will reduce a major source of income for LTC facilities.

Fifth, given these four trends, *there may be more work to do with fewer staff.* As Medicaid funding is slashed, patient turnover increases, and Medicare is dominated by managed care, LTC facilities may cut staff positions. Given a lack of authorization for mental health evaluations, a higher rate of patient turnover, and an increase in severely ill residents, staff will have to work harder and longer. Of course, this prediction has already come to pass in many nursing homes. As one administrator told us: "We've been doing more with less for years now." One exception to this trend may be LTC facilities who attract large numbers of residents with LTC insurance. Such insurance may reimburse the facilities at a higher rate than Medicare or Medicaid.

While these changes may be earth-shaking, one benefit may be an upgrading of the skills of LTC social workers and nurses. When staff have to serve more difficult patients in less time and with less consultant support, then they have to be very well-trained and versatile. Facilities will have to invest more time and money in their training, which may help staff in maintaining their morale.

CONCLUSION

While these clouds on the future horizon appear ominous, our historical overview provides us with a ray of hope: our country's advocacy groups who are determined to protect and provide for its elderly citizens. As long as that moral concern continues, we can weather the coming storm. If that commitment wanes, however, then we may lose some of the gains that we have made toward treating the whole person in LTC. What it means to treat the whole person is the topic of our next chapter.

REFERENCES

Bennett, C. (1980). *Nursing home life: What it is and what it could be.* New York: Tiresias Press.

Coleman, B. (1991). *The nursing home reform act of 1987: Provisions, policy, prospects.* Boston: Gerontology Institute, University of Massachusetts.

Davis, W. (1994). *The introduction to healthcare administration.* Bossier City, LA: Publicare Press.

German, P.S., Rouner, B.W., Burton, L.C., Brandt, L.J., and Clark, R. (1992). The role of mental morbidity in the nursing home experience. *Gerontologist, 32,* 152-158.

Health Care Financing Administration (1995). *State operations manual: Provider certification.* Washington, DC: Health Care Finance Administration. (National Technical Information Source No. PB 95950009.)

Institute of Medicine, Committee on Nursing Home Regulation (1986). *Improving the quality of care in nursing homes.* Washington, DC: National Academy Press.

Morford, T.G. (1988). Nursing home regulation: History and expectations. *Health care financing review, annual supplement,* 129-132.

Omnibus Budget Reconciliation Act of 1987, Public Law 100-203.

Subcommittee on Long-Term Care of the Special Committee on Aging, United States Senate (1974). Nursing home care in the United States: Failure in public policy, Supporting paper No. 1: The litany of nursing home abuses and an examination of the roots of controversy (Report No. 93). Washington, DC: Government Printing Office.

Chapter 2

Psychosocial Needs of LTC Residents

"The aged are not a burden . . . This is a home which is not just a place where the aged eat and sleep, but also a place where the aged can lead a life of their own." This quote from a nursing home brochure is the way that Clifford Bennett, PhD begins his 1980 book, *Nursing Home Life: What It Is and What It Could Be.* Then he makes the following comment:

> The particular rest home described above closed its doors during the mid-sixties, along with many others of its kind, to be replaced by an emerging nursing home industry that had the financial base with which to comply and cope with rapidly developing regulations for life safety, service expectations, and spiraling costs of all kinds. "Homes" gave way to "long-term care facilities" with "levels of care," language indicating a shift in physical design and service delivery modes. And with what impact on the lives of those in need of those services and facilities? (Bennett, 1980, p. 3)

This shift from "home" to "facility" in the 1960s was consistent with both the prevailing medical model and our western culture's dualistic tendency to split the mind and the body. At that time, the predominance of the medical model was reflected in the highly limited training that staff were given in the psychosocial arena. Such training was often limited to a one-hour in-service that covered needs such as dignity, safety, privacy, independence, control, and touch. Obviously, these needs are important enough to warrant more than a one-hour in-service.

In this chapter, we describe the psychosocial needs of LTC residents, using Bennett's survey as the model for such. We cite Bennett's book throughout this chapter because of the substantial influence it had when it was published, and because of the way it has shaped our own thinking. We conclude with a brief description of the Biopsychosocial Model of medicine, which is the model for assessing and treating that we use in this book.

BENNETT'S EXPERIMENT AND INFORMAL SURVEY

In response to the underemphasis upon psychosocial services in LTC, Clifford Bennett, PhD, an administrator of a 134-bed nursing home, undertook an interesting experiment in the late 1970s. Disguised as a patient, he was admitted to another nursing home to spend ten days as an "alcoholic" resident with medical problems.

Bennett provides a very moving account of his experiences there, and of the striking insights that arose from placing himself in the shoes of his residents. On the negative side, he found it humiliating to share an unlockable bathroom with others; he found it difficult to maneuver a wheelchair through doorways and around barriers; he experienced the lack of freedom as "very incarcerating;" and found it frustrating and depressing to sit in the lounge, where "the confused, the disoriented, and the incontinent were lumped together with mentally alert and rational people" (Bennett, 1980, p. 59). On the positive side, he was quite touched by the sensitive and nurturing care provided by some of the nursing staff. He gives the following account of the care he received from a nurse named Rose on his first night at the home:

> ... she pushed me over to the sink and asked if I could wash myself. I told her I could and, as I soaped and cleansed my hands, she stayed by my side and ran her hand through my hair. She was very concerned about her unkempt alcoholic charge who was spending his first night in a home. I needed this human touch and thought how beautiful it was for her to give it. Here was an example of the kindness that many nursing home staff members direct toward patients about which the general public seldom hears. (Bennett, 1980, p. 51)

When he returned to his nursing home and resumed his duties as administrator, he embarked on an extensive dialogue with his staff about the psychosocial needs of residents, using his own experience as a resident as a reference point. His premise was that when the basic human needs of residents are met, their quality of life is enhanced. In order to identify the needs that are often neglected by the medical model, he looked at differences in the scope of care rendered in LTC versus the hospital. Specifically, he made a comparative analysis of the duties and responsibilities of acute care nurses versus those working in LTC, which is reproduced in Table 2.1. Examination of this table reveals striking differences in the scope of nursing practice in the two settings.

Given that psychosocial needs are more prominent in LTC, Bennett sought to specify what these psychosocial needs are. As a starting point, he adopted Maslow's hierarchy of needs, which is shown on the left side of Table 2.2. He and his staff then listed the specific needs of LTC residents that paralleled Maslow's hierarchy, which are shown on the right side of Table 2.2.

Using these needs, Bennett developed an informal survey of his residents to determine which were most important to them. He and his staff decided that nursing homes did a good job of meeting Level I and II needs, but tended to neglect the higher needs. Thus, their survey of residents included only the 16 needs from Levels III, IV, and V. They then chose 25 of their cognitively intact residents to take the survey, which asked them to rank their needs in order of importance. The results are shown in Table 2.3, along with the way in which Bennett defined each need for the residents. We now discuss these needs in the order in which they were ranked.

1. Possessions

Much to the surprise of both Dr. Bennett and his staff, residents rated possessions as the most important need. Perhaps this should not be such a revelation, given the considerable losses experienced by LTC residents. Many of them lose their homes, cars, furniture, jobs, family, body parts, and money. In many cases, they lose all of their possessions and property, leading to a sense of destitution (Bennett, 1980).

TABLE 2.1. A Comparison of Essential Nursing Responsibilities in Nursing Homes and Acute Care Facilities

Nursing Home Nursing	*Acute Care Nursing*
Patients are served for months and years.	Patients are served for days and weeks.
Objective is to maintain the patient's well-being.	The objectives are cure oriented.
The death experience is a certainty for most patients.	Most patients are discharged to their homes.
Nurses have had long-lasting relationships with families at the time of death.	Nurse-family relationships, if any, have been relatively short at the time of death.
Nurse is involved with the patient's personal life.	Nurse is less involved with the patient's personal life.
The patients are rarely cured.	Many patients experience a cure.
High percentage of patients are dependent on nurses for their total needs.	Lower percentage of patients are dependent on nurses for their total needs.
The social and recreational needs of patients are a critical part of their care.	The social and recreational needs of patients are less significant.
The percentage of incontinent patients is high.	The percentage of incontinent patients is low.
Many mentally afflicted are served.	Few mentally afflicted patients are served.
Service is given to many non-ambulatory patients.	Most patients are ambulatory or become ambulatory.
Physicians place heavy reliance on nurses' judgment due to inconsistent physician monitoring.	Physician reliance on nurses' judgment not as great due to frequent physician monitoring.

Source: Adapted from Bennett (1980) and used by permission.

TABLE 2.2. Maslow's Hierarchy of Needs and Specific Associated Needs

Maslow's Needs	*Level*	*Specific Associated Needs*
Self-actualization	V	Accomplishment.
Self-esteem: Independence, recognition, self-respect.	IV	Freedom, privacy, independence, decision making, choice of food, choice of clothes, recognition, control over financial affairs.
Social Needs: Love belonging, affection status.	III	Family, friends, religion, possessions, communication, community involvement, purchasing.
Safety and Security Needs: Freedom from physical harm.	II	Freedom from physical harm.
Physiological Needs: food, air, drink, sleep, sex, shelter	I	Meals, drinks, sleep, sex, air, warmth, medicine, medical services.

Source: Bennett (1980). Used by permission.

Unfortunately, nursing homes are typically modeled on acute hospitals in their design, leaving little space in the small two- or three-bed rooms for personal possessions. When residents are admitted, families are asked to bring things from home, such as TVs, radios, family photos, and clothing. However, very little else is allowed because of space limitations.

The practical implication of the survey is obvious: accommodate residents' possessions whenever possible, and safeguard them. When a possession has been verified as missing, staff should act as a resident's advocate by implementing the facility's "theft and loss policy."

TABLE 2.3. Ranking of Needs by Bennett's Residents

1. *Possessions:* having one's own belongings with one.

2. *Family:* seeing one's family.

3. *Freedom:* to move about and do things.

4. *Privacy:* having the option of being alone.

5. *Independence:* doing things for oneself.

6. *Making decisions:* deciding for oneself what one wants.

7. *Choice of food:* being able to have a say about what one eats.

8. *Friends:* seeing one's friends.

9. *Choice of clothing:* having enough clothes available from which to choose what one will wear.

10. *Religion:* participating in one's religion.

11. *Control over own financial affairs:* knowledge of, and a say in, one's own financial affairs.

12. *Communication with people outside the home:* freedom to contact people outside the home.

13. *Recognition:* acknowledging one's contributions and talents.

14. *Community activities:* being involved with community life.

15. *Shopping and buying:* being able to buy things.

16. *Accomplishment:* to achieve something.

Adapted from Bennett (1980). Used by permission.

2. Families

Bennett's residents rated families as number two on the list, which reflects the great importance of family involvement for these residents. Prior to the survey, Bennett and his staff "viewed families as being motivated to visit the home and believed they would do so without special efforts" on their part (Bennett, 1980, p. 82). The survey results, however, prompted them to take a second look at how they might encourage more family support. Not only would more family visitation help the resident, it might also help family members who feel sad and guilty at having to place a loved one in a home (Bennett, 1980).

The biggest barrier to family visits is the nursing home environment, which discourages family involvement (Bennett, 1980). The standard architectural design of a nursing home often discourages visitation. The small, crowded rooms, the narrow hallways, and the absence of bedside chairs make most facilities uninviting to visitors. The lounges are crowded and have oriented and disoriented residents sitting together. Privacy is often hard to come by. When children visit, there is usually no place for them to be accommodated. Often, they become impatient and restless, and they may be asked to leave, taking their parents with them. The result is that residents may not see much of their grandchildren or great grandchildren, whom they cherish so much (Bennett, 1980).

Removing these barriers wherever possible is an important first step in encouraging greater family involvement. In addition, staff can lead a family support group to address family members' emotional distress at having to place their relative. To encourage greater involvement with the facility, they can encourage members to participate in the family council. When a resident is experiencing psychosocial or behavioral problems, a referral to the mental health consultant is often helpful, especially if she communicates her findings and treatment plan to the family. Finally, for social workers in LTC, it is imperative that they invite family members to case conferences and welcome their input.

3. Freedom

The residents' need for freedom is generally ignored and seldom discussed. Nursing homes imply at admission that residents are free to do what they want to at the time and place of their choosing, which is consistent with the "Residents' Rights" agreement. The reality is, however, that residents are "virtual prisoners," with their freedom "curbed by the physical environment" and "the outmoded care systems and procedures" (Bennett, 1980, p. 84). The architecture of homes discourages freedom of movement because there are often no "walkways, patios, exercise courses, gardens, or picnic grounds" (Bennett, 1980, p. 84). Contemporary homes have long corridors with rooms on either side, one or two lounges, and poor access to the courtyard, if there is one. As such, they lack real space for living. Other barriers to freedom are the limited staffing and the antiquated requirement that the resident have the physician's approval before going outside the home. The severely disabled are most restricted, because they are immobile and are seldom taken outside.

Not only are residents restricted physically, but on a psychological level, they feel quite alienated from the outside community. This alienation leads to the stereotyped image of residents staring out windows and parking by the doorway, hoping somehow to return to their former world. During Dr. Bennett's stay as a pseudo-patient, he observed the following interchange:

> While in the lounge one day, I overheard a disturbing verbal interchange between two patients. After gazing out of the window for a few seconds, one of them turned and said to the other, "What are we doing here?" The sad reply was, "waiting to be called!" How true it was. Admittedly, that is the regulated purpose of nursing home life. (Bennett, 1980, p. 86)

All this underscores the importance of staff's advocating for residents' freedom wherever possible. While facilities cannot be completely redesigned, staff can initiate the installation of automatic doors and make other minor changes that encourage residents to use outdoor areas. Using informed consent wherever possible enhances their sense of autonomy and control.

4. Privacy

Like freedom, privacy is virtually nonexistent. Unless residents have a private room, privacy may only be found if they "move to obscure corners, wait for their roommate to leave, or visit the lavatory" (Bennett, 1980, p. 87). Bennett points out that the curtain dividers in each room only create the illusion of privacy. They were designed for use in an acute care setting, and the implication, once again, is that what works in acute care works in LTC. Bennett notes that residents often give themselves some privacy by pulling the curtain to block the view of the person in the next bed. However, this blocks the view of the outdoors for those furthest from the window, which often leads to "arguments over who has control over the divider screens" (Bennett, 1980, p. 88).

While staff cannot change the structure of their facilities, they can respect privacy, encourage others to do so, and enforce confidentiality. Matching roommates carefully can minimize some of the common arguments over privacy.

5. Independence

Many facilities view independence as their primary objective, stressing this in staff training and striving to praise residents for doing as much as possible themselves. Unfortunately, the reality is often quite different, because understaffing and environmental factors work against independence (Bennett, 1980).

Understaffing works against independence in two ways. When few staff are available, emotionally needy residents rely on staff to do things that they themselves could do, merely for the sake of receiving attention. Often, they tie up the staff members for long periods of time. By contrast, more resilient residents, sensitive to the needs of hard-working nurses and those of the more disabled residents, often forego requests for the minor assistance that might help them to live more independently. For example, residents who need help with dressing may stay in their night clothes all day so that they do not "bother" the staff. The result is that the some of those with the greatest potential for independence are most deprived of the opportunity to achieve it (Bennett, 1980).

Concerning the impact of environment, Bennett notes that the "design and physical layout of homes play a major part in preventing patients from functioning at their maximum level" (Bennett, 1980, p. 92). For example, rooms are so congested that wheelchair patients find it very difficult to maneuver around obstacles. To get out of their room, they often need staff's assistance in moving a chair, bed, or over-the-bed table (Bennett, 1980). Finally, the layout of nursing homes often leads to crowding and "traffic jams" which restrict freedom of movement.

Staff may not be able to increase staffing levels or change the environment. However, nurses and social workers can remove barriers to mobility and independence for individual residents. By tuning in to the needs of the less vocal residents and providing attention to demanding residents only when they need it, staff can promote more independent behavior. On an environmental level, staff can make small adjustments, such as rearranging furniture, maximizing the use of common space, and removing carpet moldings at doorways.

6. Making Decisions

Bennett asks, "Do residents really have the opportunity to decide for themselves the things which affect their daily lives?" (Bennett, 1980, p. 98). Unfortunately, he answers, the opportunities are scarce because the efficient functioning of nursing homes requires the use of care schedules, routines, and care systems. At the same time, however, OBRA has mandated that staff help residents to exercise more self-determination.

Bennett points out that for many residents, their decision-making power has been removed or greatly undermined before they have even entered the nursing home. This is especially likely when cognitive impairment is involved. Many residents do not even have a choice about whether or not to go to a nursing home. Once there, they quickly become accustomed to the routine environment and their loss of decision-making power. Bennett points out that while staff often call this process "adjusting to the facility," it would be more accurately described as "conforming to the system" (Bennett, 1980).

Given these realities, what can staff do? Wherever possible, staff should encourage residents to express their individual needs and preferences. Empowerment can begin at admission, where staff can encourage residents to participate in the admissions process. If capable, they can sign their own consents, advance directives, and Residents' Rights form. With imagination and thought on staff's part, residents can be more involved with care planning, discharge planning, room placement, and the resident council.

7. Choice of Food

Eating is the only pleasurable activity for many LTC residents, and residents often look forward to the next meal as their only diversionary activity. The quality of the meals tends to be the topic most discussed in homes. Bennett believed that the general level of morale in the nursing home correlates with the residents' degree of satisfaction with the food. He also noted that family members frequently ask their relatives about its quality. If the reports are good, the family members are pleased because it reassures them that the residents are well cared for and content. Thus, for him, the home's overall image rested to a great extent upon the quality of its meals (Bennett, 1980).

Of course, choice of food is not a realistic option for most residents, unless they are fortunate enough to be in an exclusive, private facility. They can, however, have some say in the kind of food they are served. To enhance meals for residents, many facilities use dietary review panels, solicit input from the resident council, and implement social dining programs for cognitively intact residents. For less disabled residents, restaurant outings provide a refreshing break in routine and help to restore some quality of life.

8. Friends

In our discussion of families, we described barriers to their visiting; these apply to friends as well. Bennett (1980) points out that some residents compensate for the loss of old friends by developing new ones in the facility. Unfortunately, roommates are often not the ones chosen for friendship. In fact, Bennett believed that roommates are likely to distance themselves from one another, have conflicts over use of space, and be irritated by the activities and noises of the other.

To encourage old friends to visit, we offer the same suggestions as we did for families. Among the residents themselves, structured or informal activities that draw people together can help to promote friendship. Careful selection of roommates can help to minimize conflict.

9. Choice of Clothing

Bennett's residents put clothing rather low on their list, perhaps because they had "given up" on this aspect of their lives. The sad result is that in the process, another area of dignity is lost.

Sometimes, staff discourage families from bringing the resident many clothes because residents often do not leave the home. We think that this is a mistake because without their garments, residents lose a sense of self and some of their dignity. When residents can dress neatly and wear a variety of clothes, they can maintain self-respect and express their individuality.

In particular, staff should assure that each resident has an adequate selection of clothing and that the inventory is updated periodically. Since large homes have problems with lost clothes, labeling machines should be used to identify each garment. In cases where residents' families cannot provide them with what they need, community charities (e.g., Salvation Army and Jewish Family Services) may be able to help.

10. Religion

Religion's poor showing surprised Bennett, who thought that spiritual issues would be a priority for people approaching death. The poor attendance of his residents at church services supported the survey's finding (Bennett, 1980).

Bennett surmised that they did not attend because they were no longer connected with their church community. Thus, they practiced their religion primarily as individuals and not in worship services (Bennett, 1980). We would add that some do not attend because they believe that their religious faith has failed them by allowing them to end up in a nursing home. Others are simply too demented to draw strength from their religious faith.

11. Control Over Own Financial Affairs

While any loss is painful, financial loss can be especially so. However, for these residents, it was loss of possessions, not loss of financial control, that was most painful. Perhaps at this point in their lives, with all their possessions gone, they no longer yearned for financial control.

Residents on Medicaid have to live on a small monthly subsistence, which is supposed to cover clothes, toiletry items, treats, and miscellaneous items. Stretching those dollars to cover these items may prove difficult. To make matters more difficult, family members sometimes spend the money on themselves (Bennett, 1980).

It is important not to assume that residents are disinterested in financial matters. When possible, staff can empower residents in this area by giving them monthly financial statements, allowing them to control the money they do have, encouraging them to do their own shopping, and having them participate in the admissions process.

12. Communication with People Outside the Home

Residents probably rated this item low because of the obstacles to such communication. Given their disabilities, the inaccessibility of telephones, and their frequent difficulty with reading and writing, it is not surprising that they would give up on staying connected.

Staff can be creative in helping residents around these obstacles. For example, for residents who can write, family members can bring them stationery "just in case" the resident wants to use it. Community service groups, such as adult service clubs or the Girl/Boy Scouts may be available to visit or to write dictated letters. Churches formerly attended by residents can be contacted and encouraged to send visitors. Staff can also ask family members to arrange visits from community groups that the resident would enjoy.

13. Recognition

Respect and appreciation are important to all of us, so why did these residents rate it so low? We suspect that they had simply given up on gaining recognition because they were in a nursing home.

What residents can be recognized for is their past accomplishments, but these are often not known by staff (Bennett, 1980). We recommend that staff get thorough information about the residents' history, and that this information be available to other staff. In this way, staff can relate to residents' interests and can build self-esteem by acknowledging their accomplishments.

We also recommend that staff use residents' special skills in the nursing home, so that they can gain the satisfaction of making a meaningful contribution. For example, in a recent case of ours, a man who had served on the local school board was encouraged to run for president of the resident council. Similarly, residents with musical talents might perform at or help with musical activities.

14. Community Activities

Community Activities were probably rated low for the same reason as Recognition: they had little hope of achieving such in a home. Two key reasons for residents' isolation from the community are (1) that community groups tend not to maintain ties, except on a few major holidays, and (2) that nursing homes do not have the staff to take residents to community events (Bennett, 1980). Many alert, oriented residents would enjoy shopping, social events, movies, and town meetings, but homes do not provide the transportation or staff to take them there.

However, there have been some notable exceptions to this trend. One innovation has been the "adopt a grandparent" programs sponsored by elementary schools. In this program, residents go to the classroom and help with projects, with transportation sometimes provided by parents of the children. Another innovative program, set up by a nursing home, linked residents with an outside group serving the homeless, for whom the residents made sandwiches.

In looking for community groups that will come to the home, staff should search for a few well-placed contacts. Service-oriented groups, volunteer organizations, musical groups, and children's dance or gymnastics groups–all may prove receptive. If they understand the value of their contributions or that some of their former members are at the home, they may welcome the opportunity.

15 and 16. Shopping and Buying, and Accomplishment

These two areas were at the bottom of their list because residents rarely shop and often cannot accomplish much at the homes. However, in our discussion of money, we suggested that you encourage cognitively intact residents to do as much of their shopping as they can. In our discussion of recognition, we underscored the importance of learning, acknowledging, and drawing upon residents' past accomplishments and talents.

Conclusion

While nursing homes have changed considerably since Dr. Bennett's study in the late 1970s, the psychosocial needs of our elderly population remain constant. Despite the advent of OBRA and its emphasis upon the psychosocial arena, the focus of LTC continues to be Maslow's Level I (physiological) and Level II (security and safety) needs. Enhanced awareness of residents' psychosocial needs is a good start, but it is difficult to accommodate them within a poorly designed, medically oriented environment.

For this reason, Bennett created a list of 25 design specifications for a psychosocially sensitive nursing home. We have listed these "dream home" specifications at the end of this chapter. While it may be too late for established nursing homes to use these guidelines, the many assisted living centers that are now being built could adopt them.

THE BIOPSYCHOSOCIAL MODEL

Our model for this book and for our treatment in LTC is the Biopsychosocial Model. In the late 1970s, George Engel, MD, proposed that the field of medicine adopt this model. The prevailing model at that time was the biomedical model, which he considered narrow and reductionistic (Engel, 1980). In its place, Engel proposed a model based upon systems theory. Systems theory held that problems should be viewed holistically and from several different perspectives. They should not simply be broken down into parts and analyzed, as they were under the biomedical model. When he applied systems theory to medicine, Engel insisted that disease be viewed in the context of the whole person, which included not only organs and tissue, but personal experience, behavior, relationships, and culture.

This model seems intuitively obvious and correct, but it is important to realize that this holistic viewpoint was not always in vogue. Partly because of the Biopsychosocial Model, the field of medicine now lends much more weight to the influence of psychological, relational, and cultural factors upon disease. In actual practice, however, putting on our biopsychosocial eyeglasses can still be a struggle. When faced with the overwhelming medical problems of residents on a day-to-day basis, it is easy for us to slip back into the biomedical view. In the midst of a stressful workload, it takes self-discipline to look at the whole person and to address his psychosocial needs.

In this same vein, we also want to guard against being swamped by the current tide in psychiatry, which emphasizes a biological approach to treatment. We believe that the psychosocial problems of most residents demand more than a pill. Even when medication is the primary solution, assessing the whole person usually leads to other helpful interventions.

CONCLUSION

We have spent the better part of this chapter exploring the emotional and social vacuum that residents often experience in LTC. Dr. Bennett has shown us that we can do better, but it will require adopting a holistic approach and redesigning facilities. In the meantime, we have suggested ways that as individual staff members, you can meet some of these psychosocial needs.

Now that we have given you an overview of the basic psychosocial needs of residents, we will focus on more specific emotional and behavioral problems. We begin by discussing the assessment of mental and emotional disorders in the next two chapters.

SOME NURSING HOME DESIGN SPECIFICATIONS

1. A minimum of 225 square feet of floor space per bed
2. Individual four-drawer bureau for each patient
3. Armchairs and table for each patient in every room
4. Provision for television and telephone in each room
5. Clothes closet, minimum size six feet high by 30 inches deep by five feet wide, with optional locking doors
6. For each room, a private toilet with a small vanity for personal care items, minimum 48 square feet, with hand bars
7. One special family room in each unit for family visits
8. Picnic tables and fireplaces on the grounds
9. Exercise area on the grounds complete with paved walkways for strolls and wheelchairs
10. Each patient's room with a door with a centrally controlled locking device leading to the outside (optional)
11. Patio outside each patient's room (optional) or two patios for each unit

12. Lawn furniture for the patios
13. Each unit to have a minimum of two sitting rooms plus one family room and one room for congregate dining
14. All doors leading to the outside to be locked with master control for security purposes during certain hours
15. Main entrance doors to have centrally controlled television monitoring of people entering the building
16. At least one outside door of the facility which will be convenient for patients, to be opened by a centrally controlled electric eye
17. Provision for television monitoring of each patient bed
18. Innovative shower and bathing section in each unit with the following:

    • Separate dressing and undressing room, furnished with dresser and mirror, situated adjacent to the shower and bathing facilities
    • Separate bathtub room, minimum 100 square feet
    • Separate shower room, minimum 100 square feet
    • Appropriate home-like decor

19. Carpeting permitted in visitor foyer at main entrance only
20. Valuables box with locking device built into wall for each patient in every room
21. Classroom for staff education programs
22. Multiuse auditorium suitable for conversion to an ecumenical chapel
23. Mailbox for receiving mail affixed to wall outside every room for each patient
24. A main mailbox for outgoing mail in each unit
25. Play area, with swings, on grounds for children

Source: Adapted from Bennett, C. (1980). *Nursing home life: What it is and what it should be.* New York: Tiresias Press. Reprinted by permission.

REFERENCES

Bennett, C. (1980). *Nursing home life: What it is and what it could be.* New York: Tiresias Press.

Engel, G.L. (1980). The clinical application of the Biopsychosocial Model. *American Journal of Psychiatry, 137,* 535-544.

Chapter 3

Assessment of Mental Disorders in LTC

In applying the Biopsychosocial Model to psychosocial and behavioral problems, we begin with a careful assessment of the resident's mental and physical functioning. Without an initial multidisciplinary assessment, we risk plunging into interventions that may not address the most important causes of the problem. In addition, we may attempt interventions that do not account for the resident's strengths and weaknesses. For example, attempting psychotherapy with a depressed resident who has very poor recent memory may not be helpful, because the resident cannot recall what was discussed during a session. On the other hand, if that resident displayed good attention and concentration, she might be able to focus on simple activities which might elevate her mood.

When a resident presents with a psychosocial problem, we must keep in mind that the cause may be a medical one. Thus, we depend upon the resident's physician, the nurses, and therapy staff to do a careful assessment of potential physical causes. To identify the psychological and social causes of the problem, staff may be able to consult a mental health professional, such as a Licensed Clinical Social Worker, Psychiatric Nurse Consultant, Psychologist, or Psychiatrist. Of course, in some circumstances, staff have to assess the resident themselves.

In this chapter we describe the kinds of referral questions that your mental health consultant can answer, and what you should expect, in turn, from your consultant. We then discuss the key terms associated with the Mental Status Exam, an indispensable part of any mental health assessment. Finally, we describe the two most common mental disorders in LTC: cognitive impairment and depression.

Our hope is that this overview will prepare you to understand your consultant's reports, to discuss mental health issues knowledgeably with staff and your consultant, and to do better assessments by yourselves when a consultant is not available.

WORKING WITH YOUR MENTAL HEALTH CONSULTANT

If you are fortunate enough to have a good mental health consultant, you can refer many problems to him or her for assessment. The kinds of presenting problems that your consultant can assess are listed in Table 3.1.

TABLE 3.1. Presenting Problems That Your Mental Health Consultant Could Assess

- Depression or anxiety

- Delusions or hallucinations

- Verbal or physical aggressiveness

- Disruptive noisemaking

- Inappropriate sexual behavior

- Disruptive wandering

- Diagnosis of mental disorder on admission

- Admission to LTC on a psychiatric medication without a psychiatric diagnosis

- Resident's mental competency to manage money or to make medical decisions

- Resident's level of dementia

When it comes to assessing a resident, the mental health consultant should give you a written report covering several basic areas; these are listed in Table 3.2. The *history* need not be long, since much of it is in the chart, but a brief summary of the presenting problems and their recent history is helpful. While the *interview* is not always helpful if the resident is demented, the consultant should briefly describe what the resident said. The *Mental Status Exam* is essential, and its parts are discussed in the next section. While *testing* is not essential, consultants should at least use brief screening instruments for depression and dementia, such as those we describe in the next chapter. If detailed knowledge of a resident's cognitive abilities is needed, the resident should be referred to a psychologist or neuropsychologist for more testing. At the end of the evaluation, the consultant should make a psychiatric *diagnosis*, provide an answer to the referral question, and indicate what the problem's key causes are. Of course, consultants cannot always answer the referral question and identify causes, and in such cases, they should say so. If the consultant has identified causes of the presenting problems, she should provide you with specific, functional *recommendations* to use. One of the greatest deficiencies of consultants' reports is that only one or two general recommendations are made, such as for medication or psychotherapy. Such recommendations do not help staff in their day-to-day work with the resident. An example of a mental health consultant's report is provided at the end of this chapter.

One of the most important parts of the evaluation is your consultant's talking with a close family member about the resident and the

TABLE 3.2. Key Parts of a Mental Health Evaluation

- History

- Interview

- Mental Status Exam

- Testing (optional)

- Diagnosis and Summary

- Recommendations

results of the evaluation. Family members often supply very important and insightful information about the resident that is simply not available from reading the chart. Family members also find it helpful to hear the results and recommendations of the consultant's evaluation, and they often want to ask questions. Another reason for the consultant to call the family is that she is in the best position to explain her results and recommendations. LTC staff can attempt to explain these to the family by referring to the report, but the consultant usually does it best, especially when the family asks questions.

Mental health consultants are often reluctant to call the family because of the extra time involved. However, they should be able to include this in the billable time for their evaluation; usually, the call only takes five to ten minutes. In addition, since LTC staff spent time setting up the referral, the consultant should return the favor by saving them a phone call to the family. Of course, confidentiality can legitimately prevent a consultant from calling the family, in cases where a mentally capable resident objects to such communication.

THE MENTAL STATUS EXAM

The Mental Status Exam is an essential component of any Mental Health Evaluation. LTC staff should be familiar with the basic terminology of the Mental Status Exam so that they can understand their consultant's reports and so that they can do better assessments themselves.

The main parts of the Mental Status Exam are listed in Table 3.3. In the area of *appearance*, we are concerned about the person's manner of dress, grooming, and whether the person looks older or younger than her stated age. Obviously, in LTC, the resident may or may not have control over her dress and grooming. *Behavior* includes the person's level of cooperation during the interview, eye contact, degree of movement, problems with hearing or vision, and tremors or unusual movements.

There are two sides to the assessment of *emotion*: mood and affect. *Mood* refers to emotional content, whereas *affect* refers to emotional process. Mood, the emotional content, describes how someone feels, and it can be described with various labels such as "angry," "anxious," "depressed," or "euphoric." Affect, the emotional

TABLE 3.3. Components of the Mental Status Exam

- Appearance
- Behavior
- Quality of Emotion: Mood and Affect
- Quality of Thinking: Content and Process
- Cognitive Functioning

process, describes how someone generally expresses his emotion, and it can include any or all of the following: (1) the range of expressed emotion, such as "constricted" versus "full range;" (2) the appropriateness of expressed emotion; (3) the stability of emotion over time; and (4) the degree of relatedness, or face-to-face rapport, that a person displays during an interview. The term "affect" can be quite confusing, however, because many professionals use this term when discussing mood. For example, residents are often said to have "depressed affect," and mood disorders such as major depression are often called "affective disorders."

When it comes to a person's quality of *thinking*, the two main areas are *thought process* and *thought content*. Thought process refers to how well one thought is logically related to the next. This is particularly important in LTC because many demented residents display illogical thinking. Illogical thinking may involve a "tangential" thought process, in which the person talks about the relevant topic but then gradually shifts to an irrelevant one. We could liken a tangential thought process to someone traveling from New York to Seattle but ending up in Los Angeles. Illogical thinking may also involve a "circumstantial" thought process, in which the person talks about the relevant topic, then talks about an irrelevant one, and then comes back to the original topic. We could liken a circumstantial thought process to someone who is traveling from New York to Seattle by way of Dallas.

Concerning *thought content*, there are two main problems: delusions and hallucinations. Delusions are "false beliefs based on an incorrect inference about external reality" (APA, 1994, p. 765). The most common types are delusions of persecution or of reference.

In *delusions of persecution,* someone believes she is "being attacked, harassed, cheated, persecuted, or conspired against" (APA, 1994, p.766). For example, a resident may believe that a group of men are lurking around the facility waiting to abuse her in some way. In *delusions of reference*, there is the belief that "events, objects, or other persons in one's immediate environment have a particular and unusual significance" (APA, 1994, p. 765). Usually, the person thinks that the events, objects, or persons are communicating something negative or critical to him. For example, a resident watching TV news may believe that the broadcaster was personally criticizing him or warning him about something ominous. A *hallucination* is a perception without an external stimulus. The three main types are auditory (usually hearing voices), visual, and olfactory (involving the sense of smell).

Finally, a very important part of the Mental Status Exam is the assessment of cognitive functioning. The eight dimensions of cognitive functioning are listed in Table 3.4. Four of the dimensions need explanation. *Orientation* refers to whether a person understands who she is, where she is, and what the time and date are. If she knows all three, she is said to be "oriented times three." If she knows two of three, she is "oriented times two." *Construction* refers to her ability to reproduce a design or object in some way, either through drawing or putting pieces together. *Judgment* is how well a person is able to think through everyday problems and arrive at a sensible decision. *Insight* is the person's level of understanding about the causes of his emotional distress and other problems. In

TABLE 3.4. Key Dimensions of Cognitive Functioning

- Orientation
- Attention
- Language expression and comprehension
- Construction
- Recent and long-term memory
- Calculations; e.g., arithmetic problems
- Reasoning; e.g., ability to see similarities
- Judgment and Insight

the next chapter, we discuss how you can administer and interpret the Mini-Mental Status Exam, which covers most of these cognitive dimensions.

DEMENTIA, DELIRIUM, AND DEPRESSION

Now that we have given you an overview of the key components of a mental status exam, we turn to a discussion of the two most common mental problems in LTC: cognitive impairment, as manifested in dementia and delirium; and depression.

Dementia

Before we discuss dementia, it is important to distinguish between cognitive impairment and dementia. Cognitive impairment may or may not be severe enough to be called dementia. It all depends on which cognitive areas are impaired. Some patients who have bad mild head injuries or focal strokes may have very restricted cognitive impairment. These patients may be unable to recognize familiar objects (agnosia) or to name familiar objects (aphasia), yet their memory is often intact. As long as their memory is normal, we would not consider such persons to have dementia.

How many areas must be impaired before we can consider someone for a diagnosis of dementia? The answer is given in Table 3.5, which is derived from the *Diagnostic and Statistical Manual of Mental Disorders-IV* (APA, 1994). As shown here, memory and one of four other areas must be impaired before someone can be considered for a diagnosis of dementia.

Dementia used to be seen as a strictly progressive, irreversible condition. However, dementia is now viewed as having a variable course that may be "progressive, static, or remitting" (APA, 1994, p. 136). Whether dementia is progressive, static, or remitting depends upon its cause. For example, Alzheimer's dementia is always progressive, but dementia due to substance abuse could get worse, improve, or stay the same (APA, 1994). Dementia can remit completely if it is caused by problems such as depression, medications, hydrocephalus, infections, toxic conditions, or metabolic disorders (Mahler, Cummings, and Benson, 1987).

TABLE 3.5. DSM-IV Criteria for Cognitive Impairment in Various Types of Dementia

A. Impairment in recent or long-term memory.

B. One or more of the following:

   1. Aphasia (language disturbance)

   2. Apraxia (impaired ability to carry out motor activities despite intact motor function)

   3. Agnosia (failure to recognize or name objects despite intact sensory function)

   4. Impairment in executive functioning, including planning, organizing, sequencing, or using abstract reasoning.

C. These cognitive deficits cause significant impairment in social or occupational functioning and represent a significant decline from a previous level of functioning.

Source: Adapted from the *Diagnostic and Statistical Manual of Mental Disorders, Fourth Edition.* Copyright 1994, American Psychiatric Association. Used by permission.

For most readers of this book, it will come as no surprise to hear that 50 to 75 percent of residents in LTC have dementia (Curlik, Frazier, and Katz, 1991). Of these, half have Alzheimer's disease (AD) and a quarter have multi-infarct dementia (caused by multiple strokes) (Curlik, Frazier, and Katz, 1991). The remaining quarter have other types of dementia, such as those due to head trauma, Parkinson's disease, Huntington's disease, Pick's disease, or other diseases.

Alzheimer's Disease

Since Alzheimer's disease (AD) is the most common type of dementia present in nursing homes, we pause here to outline the main features of this disorder. DSM-IV lists two types of AD: early onset, which starts prior to age 65, and late onset, which starts after 65 (APA, 1994). Late onset is much more common, because the older a person gets, the more likely he or she is to contract AD. While only 2 to 4 percent of seniors over 65 have AD, the rate increases to 20 percent for those over 85 (APA, 1994). A diagnosis of AD is made by establishing that the person meets the criteria for dementia and by ruling out any other medical or psychiatric conditions that may be causing it (APA, 1994).

Concerning the course of AD, one of the first signs of the disease is poor recent memory and mildly impaired long-term memory (Cummings and Benson, 1992). From there, more and more cognitive abilities are lost each year. Reisberg's stages of progression in AD are shown in Table 3.6, along with some of the key functional losses associated with each. Note that the first stage is labeled "Possible Pre-Alzheimer's," because a substantial minority of people who exhibit these impairments do not develop Alzheimer's disease (Reisberg, 1996). For these patients, the observed deficits were probably triggered by other causes, such as "brain trauma, medical problems, or psychiatric conditions" (Reisberg, 1996, p. 416).

Concerning mental disorders that accompany Alzheimer's, about 50 percent of AD patients display delusions during the course of the disease (Cummings and Benson, 1992). Concerning depression, it is doubtful that an increased rate of depression accompanies AD, because a recent study of community-dwelling AD patients found that very few had a diagnosis of major depression (Weiner, Edland, and Luszczynska, 1994). AD patients often *appear* depressed because some of their symptoms, such as decreased energy, sleep disturbance, lack of interest, and poor concentration overlap with symptoms of depression (Cummings and Benson, 1992). These symptoms often lead caregivers to believe that their relatives are depressed when in fact they are often observing the "pseudodepressive syndrome" of AD (Weiner, Edland, and Luszczynska, 1994, p. 1008). Of course, this does not mean that AD patients never get depressed, just that AD does not appear to be a risk factor for severe depression.

Delirium

Delirium has been described as a "wandering of the mind" in which "people seem to be in a world of their own, often unable to tell whether it is night or day, what meal they have just had, and sometimes even where they are" (Schogt and Myran, 1992, p. 63).

TABLE 3.6. Stages and Levels of Impairment in Alzheimer's Disease

Stage	Estimated Duration	Example of Impaired Abilities
Possible Pre-Alzheimer's	Up to 7 years	Deteriorating job performance Difficulty with word and name finding Declining recent memory Difficulty in traveling to new locations
Mild	2 years	Increased cognitive impairment, including memory and concentration Inability to perform complex tasks of daily living, such as finances, meal preparation, and shopping
Moderate	1.5 years	Increased cognitive impairment, including very poor recent memory and some disorientation Often cannot choose clothing appropriate to the day, season, or occasion Cannot live independently
Moderately severe	2.5 years	Greater and more pervasive cognitive impairment Needs assistance with dressing, bathing, and toileting At least occasional incontinence
Severe	8+ years	Pervasive, severe cognitive impairment Early on, short phrases are spoken, verbal abilities are eventually lost Needs assistance with all ADLs Incontinent Basic psychomotor skills such as walking are eventually lost.

Source: Adapted from Reisberg (1996). Used by permission of American Psychiatric Press.

Emotionally, they may become very agitated and excited for a short time, only to become lethargic and despondent a few hours later.

The DSM-IV criteria for delirium are listed in Table 3.7. Delirium is similar to dementia in that the resident is cognitively impaired, but the symptoms of cognitive impairment differ in stability over time and quality. With reference to stability, the cognitive impairment in delirium begins suddenly and changes quickly over time, whereas in dementia, it develops slowly and is manifested in the same way over time. Qualitatively, in delirium, the ability which must be impaired is attention, an area which does not have to be impaired in dementia. Another key difference is that delirium must be caused by a medical condition, such as those listed in Table 3.8. The most common cause of delirium is "intoxication due to medications, particularly anticholinergic drugs" (Lipowski, 1989, p. 580).

Case Study 1

Schogt and Myran (1992) describe the case of a 76-year-old widow who, over a period of several days, displayed changes that were first subtle, then dramatic. At first, she began to be restless and irritable and refused to attend activities. Then the dramatic part began:

> On the third night her sleep was disrupted and she became agitated and shouted for help stating that she had seen someone at the foot of her bed. She had thrown a glass of water at this figure. Staff were able to settle her but noted that she still looked frightened and vigilant and appeared to mistake one of the staff for her deceased mother. The resident appeared improved in the morning but over the course of the day she developed a fever and began to complain of shortness of breath. She no longer recognized staff and on one occasion believed she was on a boat cruise and that the nurse handing out medication was a purser. (p. 80)

She was later transferred to the ER, where she was diagnosed with hypoxia and pneumonia. She was hospitalized, treated with antibiotics, and given Haldol (an antipsychotic) until her delirium subsided.

TABLE 3.7. DSM-IV Criteria for Delirium

A. Poor attention to environment: person cannot focus, maintain, or shift attention.

B. Deterioration in thinking, as shown by:

   1. Cognitive deficits such as poor memory, disorientation, or language disturbance, OR
   2. Perceptual disturbance such as hallucinations or delusions

C. Symptoms develop suddenly (over hours or days) and fluctuate during the course of the day.

D. Symptoms must be caused by a medical condition.

Source: Adapted from the *Diagnostic and Statistical Manual of Mental Disorders,* Fourth Edition. Copyright 1994, American Psychiatric Association. Used by permission.

TABLE 3.8. Some Major Causes of Delirium

General Causes	*Corresponding Specific Causes*
• Medication	Anticholinergic and other medications
• Insufficient blood or oxygen supplied to the brain	Heart attack, occlusion of an artery, obstruction of breathing
• Metabolic derailment	Dehydration or water intoxication, acute hypoglycemia
• Substances	Alcohol or benzodiazepine withdrawal
• Infections	Urinary tract infection, pneumonia

Source: Thienhaus, 1990.

Case Study 2

Ms. W, a cooperative 99-year-old resident, had been requesting her PRN Restoril, a sleep medication, every night for 21 consecutive nights. Then, for two nights she did not request it. On the third day, she suddenly became uncooperative, yelled at the staff, and complained of seeing "bugs on the wall." By the next day, she had recovered and displayed no further psychosis or agitation. Staff attributed her angry, psychotic episode to brief delirium caused by withdrawal from her Restoril, a benzodiazepine.

Treatment of Delirium

Given that the cause of delirium is always a medical one, the obvious treatment of choice is to address that medical problem. However, the medical treatment often takes time to work, leaving staff with a delirious resident in the meantime. In cases where the resident is extremely agitated or combative, psychiatrist Ole Thienhaus, MD, recommends "judicious administration of low doses of antipsychotic medication" which "can symptomatically contain psychotic features and secondarily reduce agitation" (Thienhaus, 1990, p. 64). Such was prescribed for the woman in the second case study.

However, Thienhaus (1990) points out that in many cases environmental interventions alone work well. He recommends that the resident be kept in a "semidark room with continuous or intermittent supervision," so that excessive stimulation can be avoided, especially the bright lights and loud noises that "can further agitate a delirious patient" (p. 64). Theinhaus points out that a completely dark room is undesirable because it may worsen psychotic symptoms. In addition, Wise and Rundell (1995) recommend that staff frequently reorient the resident to time and place and that they place a clock and calendar in the room. Wise and Rundell also emphasize that residents with hearing or visual problems should wear their glasses or hearing aids, so that they can "understand and organize the environment" (p. 42).

Differentiating Delirium and Dementia

Residents with dementia are more likely to develop delirium, "because the underlying brain disease may increase susceptibility to confusional states that may be produced by medications or other concurrent medical conditions" (APA, 1994, p. 136). Since there is cognitive impairment in both dementia and delirium, how are we to tell which a person is displaying? As the above criteria indicate, in delirium the cardinal impairment is the inability to focus or maintain attention. While the delirious resident does have memory problems, these are caused by the attention problem, not by a basic inability to recall new information. For example, if someone is not paying attention to what others tell her and what goes on around her, she has no chance at remembering anything. While demented residents also have memory problems, they usually can maintain attention for at least a very short period of time.

Another key difference is the suddenness of onset in delirium. For this reason, Schogt and Myran (1992) emphasize the importance of knowing what the resident's usual mental status and baseline cognitive functioning have been. In this way, staff can recognize an abrupt change and suspect delirium.

Case Study 3

Mr. A, a 53-year-old male with severe dementia, had displayed mild delusions of persecution for the last six years. Usually the theme of the delusions was that others were stealing his money. However, within the previous few months, his delusions had become more intense, often accompanied by yelling and striking out at staff. During these violent episodes, he often deliberately slid out of his wheelchair and sat on the floor, as a way of protecting his wallet from staff, whom he thought were trying to steal it from him. His attending physician had prescribed a PRN dose of Valium for these episodes.

He was referred to the consulting psychologist for evaluation. The psychologist noted that staff's hashmark tracking showed that he became violent only between 3 p.m. and 11 p.m. Upon psychological evaluation, he denied psychotic symptoms, including delusions, and did not appear psychotic. The next day, staff discovered that late in the day, after one of his delusional and violent outbursts, he had a very high blood sugar level. He was diagnosed with diabetes, placed on a special diet, and given medication for diabetes. His blood sugar immediately came under control, and his violent outbursts stopped abruptly. While he continued to have delusions that others were trying to steal his money, he no longer became violent or sat on the floor to protect his wallet.

Asked why, in retrospect, his violent outbursts had been restricted to the 3 p.m. to 11 p.m. shift, the Director of Nursing said that his blood sugar had probably reached its highest level during this time. By late afternoon he had eaten at least two unrestricted meals and, as was his habit, had eaten plenty of junk food during the day.

Depression

Depression is the second most common mental disorder in LTC after dementia. Studies have found that 15 to 50 percent of LTC residents have clinically significant depression, with the percentage depending upon how depression was defined (Curlik, Frazier, and Katz, 1991).

DSM-IV describes three diagnostic categories for depression: major depression, dysthymic disorder, and adjustment disorder with depressed mood. The most severe of these is major depression, and its diagnostic criteria are listed in Table 3.9. Dysthymic disorder is a milder form of depression in which the symptoms have lasted at least two years. In adjustment disorder with depressed mood, a person experiences stressful events leading to a depressed mood that exceeds what would be considered a normal reaction, given the circumstances. One large study indicated that in LTC, about 12 percent of the residents display major depression, whereas 28 percent manifest a milder depression similar to the other two diagnoses (Parmelee, Katz, and Lawton, 1989). We find that adjustment disorder with depressed mood is a common diagnosis for our residents in LTC, because their depression has been caused by recent losses associated with their LTC placement.

Two Cautions About Assessing Depression in the Elderly

We recommend that you ask residents about these symptoms of depression when you are assessing them. However, we must caution you about two issues: medical problems contributing to depression and somatic symptoms of depression associated with aging.

TABLE 3.9. DSM-IV Criteria for Major Depressive Episode

Five of the following symptoms must be present for two weeks or longer, must be severe enough to cause impairment in social/occupational functioning, must not have a physical cause (such as medications or illness), and must not be caused by grieving a recent loss:

- Depressed mood most of the day, nearly every day
- Decreased interest or pleasure in daily activities, nearly every day
- More than 5 percent weight loss or gain within one month, or decreased appetite loss or gain nearly every day
- Insomnia or hypersomnia nearly every day
- Psychomotor agitation or slowness
- Fatigue
- Feelings of worthlessness or excessive guilt
- Poor concentration or indecisiveness nearly every day
- Recurrent thoughts of death or suicide

Source: Adapted from the *Diagnostic and Statistical Manual of Mental Disorders,* Fourth Edition. Copyright 1994, American Psychiatric Association. Used by permission.

Medical Problems Associated with Depression

Both medical problems and medications are often associated with depression. Medications that can contribute to depression include antihypertensives, beta-blockers, and benzodiazepines (Wise and Rundell, 1995). Examples of medical problems associated with depression are listed in Table 3.10. These disorders may contribute to depressive symptoms in at least two ways. First, depression may be a reaction to a medical problem. For example, the losses associated with a stroke or head injury may trigger depression. Alternatively, the medical problem may lead to or exacerbate depressive symptoms. In the case of a stroke or head injury, either one could cause structural changes in the brain, which in turn might trigger biochemical changes leading to depressive symptoms.

TABLE 3.10. Examples of Medical Illnesses Associated with Depression

- *Endocrine disturbances:* diabetes mellitus, hypothyroidism

- *Viral infections:* Hepatitis, Pneumonia, Encephalitis, HIV

- *Tumors:* of the lung, pancreas, and central nervous system

- *Neurological:* Parkinson's disease, stroke, epilepsy, head injury, cerebro-vascular disease, Huntington's disease

- *Other:* hypertension, electrolyte abnormalities, anemia, alcoholism

Source: Adapted from Wise and Rundell (1995), p. 59. Used by permission of American Psychiatric Press.

It is quite difficult to figure out whether one or both of these possible causes are true for a given resident. However, the nursing staff and attending physician may wish to address the question by doing further assessment, changing medications, or observing the resident for a longer time. In some cases, the depression may resolve if the medical problem improves or the medications are changed (Wise and Rundell, 1995).

When you are assessing a given resident who has one of these medical problems, you should remember that the medical problems may be causing some of the biological symptoms of depression, including sleep disturbance, appetite or weight loss, and loss of energy (Wise and Rundell, 1995). When medical problems might be causing these symptoms, you should lend more weight to other symptoms of depression, such as "guilt, worthlessness, helplessness, hopelessness, loss of pleasure, and suicidal ideation" (Wise and Rundell, 1995, p. 57).

We should add that not only can physical problems contribute to depression, but depression can adversely impact someone's medical condition. For example, depressed residents complain of more intense pain and of more pain sites than do nondepressed residents with similar medical problems (Samuels and Katz, 1995). Those who do not eat enough become undernourished. Fatigue and lack of interest make it less likely that residents will exercise, endangering their physical conditioning.

The Aging Process and Depressive Symptoms

Not only can physical illness contribute to symptoms of depression, but the consequences of aging can mimic some of these symptoms. For these reasons, many have questioned whether somatic symptoms of depression, such as insomnia, appetite/weight loss, and fatigue are valid indicators in the elderly. A recent study looking at this issue found that appetite loss was not a valid symptom of depression in the elderly, but sleep disturbance and fatigue were (Norris, Snow-Turek, and Blankenship, 1995, p. 13). Here, fatigue was manifested by diminished levels of energy and by the feeling that "everything is an effort" (Norris, Snow-Turek, and Blankenship, 1995, p. 13). Fatigue was particularly associated with depression among the old-old LTC subjects in the study.

Does this mean that appetite and weight loss are never associated with depression in our LTC residents? Absolutely not. The study above reflects the fact that there are many causes for appetite loss in the elderly, including physical illness, the aging process, and depression. The result is that appetite loss loses the powerful association with depression that it has in younger adults. Nevertheless, there are still many LTC residents who lose appetite and weight because of depression. For this reason, residents who lose weight should be evaluated for depression when a clear physical cause cannot be identified.

Underscoring the importance of such is a study by Morley and Kraenzle, who evaluated LTC residents who had lost five or more pounds over a period of three months or more. They found that depression was the cause of weight loss for a large minority (36 percent) of the residents. For about half of the residents, it was triggered by physical causes such as cancer, a swallowing disorder, or medications (Morley and Kraenzle, 1994).

CONCLUSION

In this chapter we have emphasized depression and cognitive impairment, not only because they are so common in LTC, but also because depression and certain types of cognitive impairment are treatable. Identifying these reversible problems can make a huge difference in the mental health of our residents.

Assessing mental status, cognitive impairment, and depression is often difficult in LTC, because so many of our residents are severely disabled. Consequently, we need as many tools as possible to help us with the assessment process. We discuss two of these in the next chapter.

A MENTAL HEALTH CONSULTANT'S ASSESSMENT

Resident: Ms. D

Age: 89

Referring physician: Dr. Z

Referral: She was referred for evaluation and necessary treatment by her physician, because she has been depressed and irritable.

Assessment Procedures: Records review, consultations with Charge Nurse and Social Services Director, psychological testing, interview with client, phone interview with son, phone consultation with Dr. Z.

Background: Review of the record indicated that she is on one psychiatric medication, Restoril, 7.5 mg at bedtime PRN. She has the following medical problems: UTl, pacemaker, and left knee arthritis.

Nursing notes indicate that she has poor short-term memory. She refuses out-of-room activities and prefers to stay in bed. Her weight has been stable over the last two months. Behavioral tracking of her sleep shows that she gets seven to eight hours per night, and that staff had to give her the PRN Restoril only five times this month. Her CNA said that at times, she appears depressed and irritable, as she swears at small frustrations.

Social Services notes show that her main activity is watching TV in her room, and that she walks short distances with her walker. Her son visits regularly. She attended business college and worked as a secretary for 30 years. Her main hobby was playing the organ, which she enjoyed a great deal.

Her son said that she had been on the antidepressant Desyrel for five to six years prior to coming to the home. Dr. Z said that he had taken her off this prior to her entering the nursing home, because she was doing better emotionally. However, her son said that when she entered the home, he noticed that she became more depressed. She has never been psychiatrically hospitalized, but did have an outpatient psychiatric evaluation in the past, according to her son.

Dr. Z said that she is relatively healthy and capable of living in a less restrictive setting. The primary reason that she was admitted was that she was "afraid to go out" on her own.

Interview: Concerning her family, she said that her son visits each week, which means a great deal to her. Concerning the nursing home, she is treated well and has no complaints, except that she does not like much of the food. She would like more turkey and less pasta and rice. She said that the food is one reason she lost weight in the first several months she was here.

Concerning activities here, she enjoys eating meals in the dining hall, but is not interested in the other activities here, despite her musical interests. She prefers only to watch TV. However, she did say she would play the organ if she had one here.

Concerning mood, she is depressed and wants to die because of her having to give up her apartment and possessions. She has difficulty getting to sleep, partly because of her cough. She would like the Restoril more often, but she said that she cannot have it every night. Her appetite is poor due to her not liking the food. She cries at times because she is "just sad that I am here." She has constantly wanted to die since her admission here, though she is not suicidal. She believes her life is meaningless and there is nothing that can change this. Concerning her irritable outbursts, she admitted she has these, saying: "I've developed a temper since I've been here, which is caused primarily by frustration about having to be in a nursing home."

Psychological Testing and Mental Status Exam:

Level of Consciousness: alert

Behavior: She was lying in bed. She cooperated well and made her best effort on the testing. Because she has neither glasses nor a magnifying glass, the only visual test given on the NCSE was the Naming subtest.

Mood: moderately depressed

Geriatric Depression Scale: (orally administered)=20 (mild to moderate depression)

Affect: appropriate

Thought process: normal.

Thought content: normal; she denied hallucinations and delusions of persecution.

Cognitive Functioning, as Assessed by the Neurobehavioral Cognitive Status Exam (NCSE):

Orientation: borderline (oriented times three except for year and time of day)

Attention: average

Language Comprehension: not assessed

Language Repetition: average

Language Naming: borderline

Construction: not assessed

Recent Memory: average

Calculations: average

Abstract Reasoning: average

Judgment: average

These cognitive scores must be viewed with caution because only a brief screening instrument was used.

Diagnosis and Impressions (ICD-9 Code):

296.3 Major Depression, recurrent

She admits being depressed and tested as mildly to moderately depressed. In addition, she has a history of depression starting several years ago, for which she took an antidepressant. This antidepressant was stopped prior to her entering the home because her mood had improved. The main reason for her current depression is her having to give up her possessions and to stay here. The main behavioral manifestation of her depression is her irritable verbal outbursts. While she lost weight during her first few months at the home, her weight has stabilized over the last two months. Of particular concern is her finding no meaning in life and her constant wish that she were dead.

Cognitively, she tested as intact in all areas that could be assessed, though scores on two subtests fell on the borderline between average and mildly impaired. Staff notes indicate that she displays poor recent memory, but brief screening suggested that this is intact. Her depression may be impairing her recent memory at times.

Recommendations:

1. Given her sleep problem and depression, Dr. Z said he would consider reinstituting the Desyrel.
2. Dr. Z also recommended discussing a less restrictive placement at the care planning meeting which her son will attend later this week. If such is possible and she wants to do so, it might help to relieve some of her depression.
3. If she stays at the home, I recommend a trial of weekly psychotherapy with D.L., PhD, to address her depression. Hopefully, the therapy may help her to find some meaning in her life if she stays here.
4. She said she does not like some of the food, such as the rice and pasta. Staff may wish to evaluate her preferences in this regard.
5. She said she would play the organ if one were available, but she has no glasses for reading sheet music. The Activities staff may wish to explore ways to help her participate in musical activi-

ties, or perhaps assist her in playing the piano or an electric keyboard.

6. Wherever possible, staff should ignore her irritable outbursts and approach her when she is calm.

REFERENCES

American Psychiatric Association (1994). *Diagnostic and statistical manual of mental disorders,* fourth edition. Washington, DC: American Psychiatric Association.

Cummings, J.L. and Benson, D.F. (1992). *Dementia: A clinical approach.* Boston: Butterworth-Heinemann.

Curlik, S.M., Frazier, D., and Katz, J.R. (1991). Psychiatric aspects of long-term care. In J. Sadavoy, L. Lazarus, and L. Jarvik (Eds.), *Comprehensive Review of Geriatric Psychiatry* (pp. 547-564). Washington, DC: American Psychiatric Press.

Lipowski, Z.J. (1989). Delirium in the elderly patient. *The New England Journal of Medicine,* 320, 578-582.

Mahler, M.E., Cummings, J.L., and Benson, D.F. (1987). Treatable dementias. *Western Journal of Medicine,* 146, 705-712.

Morley, J.E. and Kraenzle, D. (1994). Causes of weight loss in a community nursing home. *Journal of the American Geriatrics Society,* 42, 583-585.

Norris, M. P., Snow-Turek, A.L., and Blankenship, L. (1995). Somatic depressive symptoms in the elderly: Contribution or confound? *Journal of Clinical Geropsychology,* 1, 5-17.

Parmelee, P.A., Katz, J.R., and Lawton, M.P. (1989). Depression among the institutionalized age: Assessment and prevalence estimation. *Journal of Gerontology,* 44, M22-29.

Reisberg, B. (1996). Alzheimer's disease. In J. Sadavoy, L.W. Lazarus, L.F. Jarvik, and G.T. Grossberg (Eds.), *Comprehensive Review of Geriatric Psychiatry II* (2nd Edition*).* Washington, DC: American Psychiatric Press.

Samuels, S.C. and Katz, IB. (1995). Depression in the nursing home. *Psychiatric Annals,* 25, 419-424.

Schogt, B. and Myran, D. (1992). Delirium. In D.K. Conn, N. Herrmann, A. Kaye, D. Rewilak, A. Robinson, and B. Schogt (Eds.), *Practical psychiatry in the nursing home* (pp. 63-85). Seattle: Hogrefe and Huber.

Thienhaus, O.J. (1990). Delirium. In D. Bienenfeld (Ed.), *Clinical geropsychiatry* (pp. 59-65). Baltimore: Williams and Wilkins.

Weiner, M.F., Edland, S.D., and Luszczynska, H. (1994). Prevalence and incidence of major depression in Alzheimer's disease. *American Journal of Psychiatry,* 151, 1006-1009.

Wise, M.G. and Rundell, J.R. (1995). *Consultation psychiatry* (second edition). Washington, DC: American Psychiatric Press.

Chapter 4

The Geriatric Depression Scale
and Mini-Mental State Exam

While it would be nice to have a mental health consultant available to evaluate all new admissions to LTC, Medicare does not pay for screening. Furthermore, not all LTC facilities have mental health consultants, and even when they do, managed care companies or attending physicians sometimes refuse to authorize their services. For these reasons, social workers and nurses must often do their own version of an abbreviated mental status exam. Since cognitive impairment and depression are the two most common mental problems in LTC residents, it is most important to assess these two areas.

Fortunately, there are two instruments that can help you to screen residents in these areas. The Geriatric Depression Scale (GDS) is a very brief depression scale for the elderly, and the Mini-Mental State Exam (MMSE) is an effective dementia-screening instrument. In this section we describe each instrument, and teach you how to administer, score, and interpret it. We then relate these scores to the corresponding sections in the Minimum Data Set (MDS).

THE GERIATRIC DEPRESSION SCALE

When it comes to assessing depression in LTC, the Geriatric Depression Scale (Yesavage et al., 1983) is the measurement tool of choice for two reasons. First, it is as accurate as the mostly widely used instrument, the Beck Depression Inventory, in detecting depression among the elderly (Norris et al., 1987; Olin et al., 1992). Second, there are practical advantages in using the Geriatric Depression Scale (GDS) with an LTC population, such as ease of comprehension and ease of oral administration. The "yes/no" format of the questions is easier for the residents to understand, as compared to multiple choice formats.

While the GDS is an effective screening instrument for elderly persons without dementia, caution must be used when it is given to those with dementia. Studies evaluating its accuracy in diagnosing depression in demented elders have shown mixed results (Lichtenberg, 1994). Some studies show poor agreement between GDS scores and interview-based assessments of demented persons, whereas others have shown good agreement between the two. Given these results, we should not rely strictly on the GDS for our conclusions about a demented resident's level of depression. As we discussed in the last chapter, you should supplement your assessment of a resident's mood with reports from nursing staff and family members.

Administering the GDS

The GDS is presented at the end of this chapter. Reading the items to the resident is usually necessary because many residents are incapable of reading or tend to skip lines when reading and marking items. Before reading the items to the resident, you should begin with the instructions, "I am going to read you some questions and I would like you to respond 'yes' or 'no', based upon how you have felt over the last week." In cases where you are uncertain whether to administer it orally or to have the resident self-administer it, you can ask his preference. If he chooses to self-administer it, you can then watch to see if he is having problems. For residents who speak little or no English, you will need to use an interpreter or have a staff member who is fluent in that language administer the test.

Because the GDS was not developed exclusively for a LTC population, two of the items seem awkward. Most people admitted to a LTC facility must say "yes" to item 2, "Have you dropped many of your activities and interests?" Item 12 appears irrelevant to someone in a LTC facility: "Do you prefer to stay at home, rather than going out and doing new things?" For residents who are confined to the facility, you can rephrase this question, "Do you prefer to stay *here in your room*, rather than going out and doing new things?" For residents who frequently go out of the facility, you can phrase this question, "Do you prefer to stay *here at the nursing home*, rather than going out and doing new things?"

Sometimes residents forget to answer "yes" or "no," preferring to comment on the item or to tell a story. In that case, it is sometimes obvious that the answer is affirmative or negative. In other cases, you should repeat the item and ask for a "yes" or "no" answer. Sometimes it is clear that the resident cannot decide, or is unwilling to give a clear answer, in which case you can skip that question.

Keep in mind, however, that anytime you skip an item, you risk getting an artificially low score. The cutoff score for depression was developed with the assumption that examinees would respond to all items. Someone who does not respond to five items may have just lowered his score on the test by as many as five points. For this reason, it is best to attempt to score each item "yes" or "no." If then you cannot score nine or more items, you should not use the score as a valid index of the resident's depression (Yesavage, June 26, 1996, personal communication).

Scoring and Interpreting the GDS

The GDS is scored by adding up the number of items for which a capitalized "YES" or "NO" has been circled. When a capitalized response is circled, it means that the resident responded to the item in the depressed direction rather than the nondepressed direction. The score ranges from 0 to 30.

The resident's level of depression can be interpreted as depicted in Table 4.1. As we mentioned above, if the resident is demented, this score must be viewed more cautiously. While it is usually a good idea to interview family members and caregivers about a resident's mood, this is especially important in the case of residents with dementia. If a contradiction emerges between the resident's self-report on the GDS and the report of others, you may need to observe the resident for a longer time to resolve the issue.

Caution also needs to be used when you get a nondepressed score from a man who is showing some signs of depression. One study found that depressed men were less likely than depressed women to score above the cutoff score of 11 on the GDS (Allen-Burge et al., 1994). The authors of the study speculate that "perhaps older men are less likely to admit some feelings associated with depression because

TABLE 4.1. Scores and Levels of Depression for the GDS

Score Range	Level of Depression
0-10	Not depressed
11-20	Mildly depressed
21-30	Moderately to severely depressed

Source: Yesavage et al., 1983.

of long-term sex-role socialization" (p. 445). Once again, the implication is that you should use all sources of information to arrive at a conclusion about a person's level of depression.

To reiterate, scores cannot be taken as proof that a resident is depressed or not. No test is 100 percent accurate. You should treat the GDS score not as a conclusion, but as a hypothesis about the resident's mood that calls for ongoing evaluation.

Responding to GDS Scores

When a resident scores as depressed on the GDS, you should consider referring the resident for evaluation by your mental health consultant. Even if the person has a diagnosis of depression and is taking antidepressant medication, an evaluation of her present depression is often helpful. The consultant may find that there has been no improvement since the person started taking the antidepressant, or that additional interventions are needed.

In some cases, a resident with a diagnosis of depression tests as not depressed. Here again, this is an opportunity for your consultant to clarify what is going on. It may be that the person is no longer depressed and does not need continued treatment for depression. On the other hand, your consultant may find that the person is minimizing her depression while other evidence points to its presence. In other cases, a resident might not be currently depressed but may have a very long history of depression, making it imperative that you continue efforts to prevent another depressive episode.

In instances where you do not have a mental health consultant available, it is helpful to interview the resident about symptoms of depression that are not covered by the GDS. In Table 4.2, we have listed four of these symptoms and the corresponding questions that you can ask the resident. Of course, the reason that appetite loss, insomnia, and low energy are not assessed by the GDS is that they can be caused by medical problems, not just depression. Thus, you must be cautious about assuming that these three symptoms are caused strictly by depression. In addition to interviewing the resident, you should also get the family's reading on the person's mood. You can then discuss your findings at your care-planning meetings.

TABLE 4.2. Supplementary Questions for Assessing Depression

DSM-IV Symptom of Major Depression	Questions
• Appetite loss	"Are you hungry at mealtime?"
• Insomnia	"How well do you sleep? Do you have trouble getting to sleep or staying asleep?"
• Fatigue	"Do you feel tired much of the time, or do you have a good amount of energy? Does everything seem to take too much effort?"
• Thoughts of death or suicide	"Do you ever wish you were dead? (If so) have you ever thought about hurting yourself? (If so) what have you thought about doing?"

THE MINI-MENTAL STATE EXAMINATION (MMSE)

Developed by Folstein, Folstein, and McHugh in 1975, the Mini-Mental State Exam (MMSE) is the most commonly used cognitive screening instrument. Studies have shown that the MMSE accurately identifies people with dementia, especially when their dementia is moderate to severe in nature (Lezak, 1995).

The MMSE is a structured way of covering the cognitive part of the Mental Status Exam which we discussed earlier. Most of the key aspects of intellectual functioning are briefly tested, including orientation, recent memory, attention, calculation, and language. A major advantage is that administration takes only five to ten minutes, a length of time easily tolerated by most LTC residents. The MMSE and instructions for administration are presented at the end of this chapter.

Note that the exam covers five of the major cognitive dimensions that we listed in Table 3.4 of the last chapter. The first ten questions assess *orientation*. *Attention* is assessed through serial 7s or by spelling "world" backwards (items 3a and 3b). Recent *memory* is addressed by the three-word recall (item 4). *Language comprehension* and *expression* are assessed through naming objects (item 5a), repeating a phrase (item 5b), obeying a three-stage oral command (item 5c), obeying a written command (item 5d), and writing a sentence (item 5e). *Construction* is assessed by having the resident copy intersecting pentagons (item 5f).

Administering and Scoring the MMSE

Instructions for the MMSE have been integrated into the exam, question by question. Note that you do need a few materials to give the test, including a pencil, a watch, a blank piece of paper, and a paper with two intersecting pentagons drawn on it and the phrase "CLOSE YOUR EYES" written on it. Before administering it to an actual resident, you should practice giving it to a colleague or friend. In this way, your first few administrations will go more smoothly.

Disabled Residents

Note that some disabled residents cannot take all the test items. For example, residents who cannot write or draw cannot take items 5e and 5f, Writing and Construction. Blind residents cannot take any of the Language items except Repetition (5b).

It is extremely important to have the resident wear a hearing aid or glasses if they are prescribed. For this reason, we have provided a place at the beginning of the test to mark if the resident was wearing these. Sometimes the resident cannot wear the prescribed device at the time of testing because it is broken or cannot be found. In those cases, you would ideally delay testing until the device is available. However, when such is not feasible, you should pay close attention to the resident's nonverbal cues in order to determine if they are hearing or seeing accurately. Hearing-impaired residents who repeatedly ask you to repeat questions probably cannot be validly tested. For visually impaired residents without glasses, you may need to write the phrase, "CLOSE YOUR EYES" in extra large letters. For these people, drawing the pentagons may prove very difficult because even if they see the design, they may not be able to see their own drawing very well. Similarly, writing a sentence may prove difficult. You will simply have to use your judgment about whether it was a fair test of their ability to write or draw a design. If you decide it was not a fair test, you can decide not to score those items. Wherever possible, of course, you should administer every item, because the test was created using subjects who completed all items.

Residents who cannot use both hands are not able to complete the three-step command of item 5c. For such residents, you should give a three-step command that does not involve the use of both hands, such as: "Raise your hand above your head, touch your nose, and look at the ceiling."

Language Problems

Many of our residents did not learn English as a first language, and thus a low score from them may not reflect intellectual impairment as much as poor comprehension of your instructions. In these cases, it is often helpful to talk with the family about how fluent the resident is in English. You can then decide whether to administer it in English or to use a translator, such as a family or staff member. Of course, if you are fluent in the resident's language, you can write the exam in that language or obtain a copy of the MMSE in that language.

In some cases, residents with dementia revert to speaking only their first language, even though they were fluent in English at one point in their lives. In these cases, translation is usually necessary.

If you give the exam in a different language or use a translator, the content of two of the items will change. On the alternative Attention task (3b), you will need to substitute a five-letter word in their language. On the language Repetition task (5b), you will need to substitute a different phrase that is similar in length. For example, the Spanish version of the MMSE uses "mundo" (world) for item 3b and the phrase, "No hay pero que valga," for item 5b. Be sure to write out the phrase, "CLOSE YOUR EYES," in that resident's language prior to starting the exam.

When you decide to give the exam in English to a bilingual resident, you will have to decide as you give the exam whether or not the resident comprehends your questions. You will usually get a good sense of this on the Orientation questions. If the resident gives no response or keeps asking that the question be repeated, you should use a translated version.

Scoring

You score the MMSE by totaling the points from each section or item. The total score ranges from 0 to 30. We do not advise using the total MMSE score in residents for whom you must skip items constituting more than two possible points. Rather, you can look at how well the person did on individual items and apply these findings to the Minimum Data Set (MDS) and the treatment plan.

When Does an MMSE Score Lie in the Impaired Range?

When a person scores 23 points or fewer out of the 30 possible points on the MMSE, his/her score lies in the cognitively impaired range (Crum et al., 1993). However, this cutoff score should not be used with everyone, especially in LTC, because education and age play an important role in how someone performs on the exam. The older and less educated someone is, the lower that person tends to score on the test (Crum et al., 1993). The reverse also holds, as younger and more highly educated people score higher on the MMSE (Crum et al., 1993). An older, poorly educated person who scores 23 points or less may be giving us a false reading of cognitive impairment. Similarly, a highly educated person scoring 24 points or more may be giving us a false reading of average cognitive functioning. For these reasons, it is wise to compare an individual's score with that of others of similar age and education.

Thus, we have provided cutoff scores based on age and education in Table 4.3. The scores were calculated using data provided by Crum et al. (1993), who surveyed over 18,000 adults living in the community. We calculated cutoff scores that lie at least 1.5 standard deviations below the mean, which is about the ninth percentile. We designated these scores as constituting the beginning of the "cognitively impaired range".

Before determining which reference group to use for a given resident, you should make sure you have accurate information about his or her level of education. Family members often provide more accurate information about this than the resident. In cases where the resident has a year or less of business, technical, or trade school, you should not count this as a thirteenth year of education. These individuals should be considered as having 9 to 12 years of education.

TABLE 4.3. Recommended Cutoff Scores for Cognitive Impairment on the MMSE

Years of Education	Age Range	Cutoff Score
0-4	40-74	19
	75-79	18
	80-84	16
	85+	14
5-8	40-74	23
	75-84	22
	85+	18
9-12	40-79	23
	80+	21
13+	40-69	26
	70+	25

Source: Cutoff scores were derived from norms provided by Crum et al. (1993).

Once you are sure of the resident's educational level, you can determine whether or not it falls into the impaired range by simply finding the age and educational category and looking at its corresponding cutoff score. If the score is *equal to or less than* the cutoff score, the person has tested as cognitively impaired. If the score is *greater than* the cutoff score, then the person has tested as not impaired.

In cases where you skipped or decided not to score MMSE items totaling one or two possible points, you should lower the cutoff score by the total possible points for those items. For example, if you skipped items 5e (one point) and 5f (one point) for a 79-year-old high school graduate, you would lower the cutoff from 23 to 21. In cases where you skipped items totaling 3 points or more, we do not recommend that you adjust the cutoff score by lowering it by the number of items skipped. In these cases, you should use the information obtained on individual items, but not try to rate the person's overall level of cognitive impairment. We recommend this because the cutoffs were derived from studies in which each person took the whole exam.

Cautions About MMSE Scores

Since many of our readers may not have formal training in the use of tests, we offer four basic cautions about the use of MMSE scores. First, all tests misclassify at least a small percentage of people. Despite its good track record, the MMSE can do so also. Some individuals who score above the cutoffs are cognitively impaired, and some who score below the cutoffs are not cognitively impaired. That is why it is important to integrate the test score with other observations and sources of information, and perhaps to get a second opinion from your mental health consultant.

A second caution concerns the possible instability of MMSE scores. Because the cognitive functioning of residents in LTC often fluctuates from day to day, a resident who scores as impaired one day can score as intact the next. If a resident's intellectual ability seems to vary from day to day, it is often a good idea to administer the exam on different days, in order to get a sense of how much it varies.

Third, even when someone consistently scores as cognitively impaired on the MMSE, that result alone should not lead us to a definitive diagnosis of dementia. The MMSE cannot be used as the sole method in diagnosing dementia, because as we pointed out in the last chapter, there are a number of criteria for diagnosing dementia. Your multidisciplinary staff should use the score as only one piece of evidence for dementia. Other issues, such as whether the person displays social and functional incompetence, are equally important.

Finally, when someone gets all the items correct on the MMSE, it is important to remember that this does not mean that the person is particularly intelligent. This test simply tells us about the likely presence or absence of cognitive impairment, not about someone's IQ.

Responding to MMSE Scores

Having a resident score in the impaired range on the MMSE is no surprise, since we know that 50 to 70 percent of LTC residents are demented. In fact, we expect impaired scores from residents who have been admitted with diagnosed neurological problems or dementia. In these cases, an impaired score is no surprise and further evaluation is usually not necessary.

However, action is required in two circumstances: (1) the resident has an impaired MMSE score but has no diagnosis of dementia or neurological problems, or (2) the resident has a normal MMSE score but has a diagnosis of dementia or neurological problems. In these cases, you should refer the resident to your mental health consultant or a psychologist for further evaluation.

When a normal MMSE score is obtained from a resident with a diagnosis of dementia, it may be that the diagnosis was made erroneously because it was based upon limited information. Further evaluation might show that the person's cognitive impairment was transient or not as severe as once thought. In cases where the resident has a well-documented neurological problem, such as a stroke or Parkinson's disease, the impairment may be so mild that it cannot be considered dementia.

When a resident without neurological problems or a diagnosis of dementia scores in the impaired range, further evaluation is essential. The score may reflect a change in the resident's health, such as a new stroke or delirium. To verify the decreased cognitive ability, you could refer the person for psychological testing to learn more about the nature of the cognitive impairment. You could also refer him for a neurological or other medical evaluation to identify the underlying cause.

Finally, we should mention a puzzling situation that sometimes occurs. Occasionally, a highly educated resident scores above the recommended MMSE cutoff, even though her behavior suggests that her cognitive abilities have declined. This is particularly likely to occur in cases where the resident has mild dementia (Galasko et al., 1990). In these cases, the resident may in fact have suffered a decline in abilities, but her intellectual attainment started at such a high level that a simple test like the MMSE cannot identify the impairment. Staff should refer the resident to their consultant or a psychologist, who can provide more adequate testing and further evaluation.

In cases where a consultant or psychologist is not available or further assessment is not authorized, you will have to discuss these findings in your interdisciplinary meetings and consult with the attending physician. Discussing the MMSE score at your meetings has practical value, in that you will have informed staff about what cognitive level to expect from this resident. By discussing your findings with the attending doctor, you will have covered yourself from a legal standpoint because the physician is the one most responsible for identifying the resident's medical diagnoses.

APPLICATION OF FINDINGS TO THE MDS 2.0

These two instruments can help you to complete two sections of the MDS (Minimum Data Set) 2.0 more accurately: Section E, "Mood and Behavior Patterns," and Section B, "Cognitive Patterns." We now discuss specifically how the GDS and the MMSE can be applied to the completion of these sections.

Application of GDS Scores to the MDS 2.0, Section E

Section E of the MDS 2.0, takes a behavioral approach to assessing depression. In Part 1 of this section, you are to rate how frequently the resident displays behavioral "indicators of depression, anxiety, and sad mood," including "verbal expression of distress"; "sleep-cycle issues"; "sad, apathetic, anxious appearance"; and "loss of interest."

While many of these items can be rated based upon observation, the resident's answers to individual GDS items can help you to rate some of these items. Question 17 asks, "Do you feel pretty worthless the way you are now?" which is relevant to item e, "self depreciation." Question 8 asks, "Are you afraid that something bad is going to happen to you?" which applies to MDS item g, "statements that something bad is about to happen." Question 27 asks, "Do you enjoy getting up in the morning?" which applies to MDS item j, "unpleasant mood in the morning." Question 13 asks, "Do you frequently feel like crying?" which helps to answer item m, "crying, tearfulness." These MDS items and the corresponding GDS questions are listed in Table 4.4.

The GDS is most helpful in answering Part 3, "Change in Mood." Here, you can repeat the administration of the GDS after 90 days, and compare this score with the previous one. Of course, this rating should not be based solely on the GDS score, but hopefully, it will be consistent with the behavioral ratings that you make in Part 1. If the GDS indicates one trend and the behavioral ratings another, there might be three reasons for this: (a) the GDS score is an inaccurate reflection of the resident's mood; (b) the behavioral observations have been inaccurate; or (c) the resident's behavioral signs of distress are not related to depression, but to some other problem, such as pain, anxiety, or delirium/dementia. Your multidisciplinary team may have to do a critical reevaluation of the resident, or refer him for an evaluation by your mental health consultant.

TABLE 4.4. GDS Questions Corresponding to Items on the MDS 2.0

Item from MDS 2.0. Section E. Part 1	GDS Question
e. "self depreciation"	17
g. "statements that something bad is about to happen"	8
j. "unpleasant mood in the morning"	27
m. "crying, tearfulness"	13

Applying the MMSE to the MDS 2.0, Section B

Because the MDS 2.0 is behaviorally oriented, Section B does not ask for a global rating of the resident's cognitive functioning. Rather, it asks whether a resident is impaired in certain areas and about specific behaviors indicative of "delirium-periodic disordered thinking/awareness." Individual items from the MMSE are helpful in rating these items.

Section B, Part 2a asks about short-term memory over a five-minute period. Such could be scored as impaired if the resident recalled only zero or one of the three words on item 4 (Recall) of the MMSE. Section B, Parts 3a and 3d ask about whether the resident knows the "current season" and "that he/she is in a nursing home," respectively. These items can be checked if the resident answered these questions correctly on MMSE items 1a and 1b, Orientation to Time and Orientation to Place. Section B, Part 5a of the MDS asks if the resident is "easily distracted," which can be answered by referring to the resident's performance on the Attention item of the MMSE (3a or 3b). If the resident scored three or fewer points on this task, you could rate the resident's attention as impaired. Of course, whether you scored it a "1" or "2" would depend upon your knowledge of the resident's past functioning. These MDS items and the corresponding MMSE questions are summarized in Table 4.5.

Section B, Part 6 asks if the resident's cognitive status has changed over the last 90 days. Here, repeated administration of the MMSE every 90 days will help you to answer this question.

TABLE 4.5. MMSE Items Corresponding

Item from MDS 2.0. Section B	MMSE Item
2a. Short-term memory	4
3a. Current season	1a
3d. That he/she is in a nursing home	1b
5a. Easily distracted	3a or 3b

CONCLUSION

Using these two tools in your assessments will not always lead to clear-cut conclusions. They are simply screening instruments designed to give you a rough estimate of a resident's level of depression and cognitive functioning. However, getting that estimate can lead to important hypotheses about a resident's problems, which can then be further explored. If those hypotheses are confirmed, staff can develop an effective treatment plan. In cases where residents are depressed, this plan may involve counseling, which is the topic of our next chapter.

THE GERIATRIC DEPRESSION SCALE

Directions: Choose the best answer for how you felt over the last week.

1. Are you basically satisfied with your life? yes/NO
2. Have you dropped many of your activities and interests? YES/no
3. Do you feel that your life is empty? YES/no
4. Do you often get bored? YES/no
5. Are you hopeful about the future? yes/NO
6. Are you bothered by thoughts you can't get out of your head? YES/no
7. Are you in good spirits most of the time? yes/NO
8. Are you afraid that something bad is going to happen to you? YES/no
9. Do you feel happy most of the time? yes/NO
10. Do you often feel helpless? YES/no
11. Do you often get restless and fidgety? YES/no
12. Do you prefer to stay at home, rather than going out and doing new things? YES/no
13. Do you frequently worry about the future? YES/no
14. Do you feel you have more problems with memory than most? YES/no

15. Do you think it is wonderful to be alive now? yes/NO

16. Do you often feel downhearted and blue? YES/no

17. Do you feel pretty worthless the way you are now? YES/no

18. Do you worry a lot about the past? YES/no

19. Do you find life very exciting? yes/NO

20. Is it hard for you to get started on new projects? YES/no

21. Do you feel full of energy? yes/NO

22. Do you feel that your situation is hopeless? YES/no

23. Do you think that most people are better off than you are? YES/no

24. Do you frequently get upset over little things? YES/no

25. Do you frequently feel like crying? YES/no

26. Do you have trouble concentrating? YES/no

27. Do you enjoy getting up in the morning? yes/NO

28. Do you prefer to avoid social gatherings? YES/no

29. Is it easy for you to make decisions? yes/NO

30. Is your mind as clear as it used to be? yes/NO

Source: Yesavage et al. (1983). Development and validation of a geriatric depression screening scale: A preliminary report. *Journal of Psychiatric Research*, 17, 37-49. Reprinted by permission of Elsevier Press.

THE MINI-MENTAL STATE EXAM

Resident _____

Age _____

Years of Education _____

Examiner _____

Date _____

If resident has glasses, these were ___worn ___ not worn.

If resident has a hearing aid, this was ___worn ___ not worn.

Instructions: Be sure the resident is wearing glasses or a hearing aid if he has them. Say to the resident, "I'm going to ask you some routine questions. Some will be difficult, while others will be easy. Just try to answer each question as best you can."

1. a. *Orientation to Time*

Item	Question	Points (0 or 1)
Year:	What *year* is it now?	_____
Season:	What is the *season*?	_____
Day of month:	What is today's *date*?	_____
Day of week:	What is the *day* of the *week*?	_____
Month:	What *month* is it?	_____

1. b. *Orientation to Place*

Item	Question	Points (0 or 1)
State:	What *state* is this?	_____
County:	What is the name of this *county*?	_____
City:	What is the name of this *city*?	_____
Building:	What is the name of this *building*?	_____
Floor:	What *floor* are we on?	_____

Total Points for Orientation (0-10): _____

2. *Registration*:

Tell the resident, "I'm going to say the names of three common objects. Just listen and say them back to me: BALL, FLAG, TREE."

Score number recalled on first trial (0-3 points): _____

If the resident did not repeat all three objects correctly on the first trial, keep reciting them to the resident and having her repeat them back to you. Do this until the resident repeats them correctly, or until you have given the resident six trials.

3. a. *Attention:Serial 7s*

Say to the resident, "I'd like you to start at 100 and count backwards by 7s. Begin with 100, take away seven, then take away seven from that, and keep taking away seven until I say 'stop'."

Check which correct responses the resident makes and score one point for each:

93 _____86 _____79 _____72 _____65 _____

Score (0-5): _____

3.b. *Alternative Attention Test*

If the resident cannot or will not perform the Serial 7s task above, ask him to spell the word, "WORLD" backwards. The score is the number of letters in correct order; e.g., dlrow= 5, dlorw= 3. Fill in the score above in place of the Serial 7s score.

4. *Recall*

Ask the resident, "Remember the three words I read to you a moment ago? Tell me the three words now." Check the words recalled:

Ball _____Flag _____Tree _____

Score (0-3): _____

5. a. *Language: Naming*

Show the resident a *pencil* and say, "Tell me the name of this object." Repeat this for a *wristwatch*.

Score one point for each item. Score (0-2): _____

5. b. *Language: Repetition*

Say: "Repeat after me: NO IFs, ANDs, OR BUTs." Allow only one trial.

Score (0-1): _____

5. c. *Language: Three-Stage Command*

Place a 8.5″ by 11″ sheet of paper in front of the resident and say, "Take this paper in your right hand, fold the paper in half, and put it on the floor." Check which parts he/she does correctly and score one point for each.

Takes paper in right hand _____   Folds in half_____

Puts on floor _____

Score (0-3): _____

5. d. *Language: Reading*

Give the resident a blank piece of paper with the sentence, "CLOSE YOUR EYES" written on it in large letters. Say: "Please read this and do what it says." Score one point if the resident closes her eyes.

Score (0-1): _____

5. e. *Language: Writing*

Give the resident a pen or pencil and sheet of paper. If the resident is lying in bed, have the paper on a clipboard or use the bed table. Say: "Write a complete sentence here [pointing]. It can be anything you want, but make sure it's a *complete* sentence." Give one point credit for any product that has a subject and verb and makes sense.

Score (0-1): _____

5. f. *Language: Copying*

Have the resident keep the paper and pen or pencil for the moment, but turn over the paper so that a clean side is exposed. Give the resident a page with intersecting pentagons of 1 to 5 cm per side (see illustration below). Say: "Copy these exactly as you see them here." Give one point credit if each figure has five angles and the two figures intersect.

Score (0-1): _____

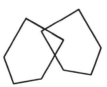

Total MMSE Score: _____

Score suggests:
_____ No cognitive impairment   _____ Cognitive Impairment

Note: Adapted from Folstein, Folstein, and McHugh (1975). Oxford: Elsevier Press. Reprinted by permission.

REFERENCES

Allen-Burge, R., Storandt, M., Kinscherf, D.A., and Rubin, E.H. (1994). Sex differences in the sensitivity of two self-report depression scales in older depressed inpatients. *Psychology and Aging*, 9, 443-445.

Crum, R.M., Anthony, J.C., Bassett, S.S., and Folstein, M.F. (1993). Population-based norms for the Mini-Mental State Examination by age and educational level. *Journal of the American Medical Association*, 269, 2386-2391.

Folstein, M.F., Folstein, S.E., and McHugh, P.R. (1975). "Mini-Mental State": A practical method for grading the cognitive state of patients for the clinician. *Journal of Psychiatric Research*, 12, 189-198.

Galasko, D., Klauber, M.R., Hofstetter, R., Salmon, D.P., Lasker, B., and Thal, L.J. (1990). The Mini-Mental State Examination in the early diagnosis of Alzheimer's disease. *Archives of Neurology*, 47, 49-52.

Lezak, M.D. (1995). *Neuropsychological assessment*. New York: Oxford.

Lichtenberg, P.A. (1994). *A guide to psychological practice in geriatric long-term care*. Binghamton, New York: The Haworth Press.

Norris, J.T., Gallagher, D., Wilson, A., and Winograd, C.H. (1987). Assessment of depression in geriatric medical outpatients: The validity of two screening measures. *Journal of the American Geriatrics Society*, 35, 989-995.

Olin, J.T., Schneider, L.S., Eaton, E.M., Zemanky, M.F., and Pollock, V.E. (1992). The Geriatric Depression Scale and the Beck Depression Inventory as screening instruments in an older adult population. *Psychological Assessment*, 4, 190-192.

Yesavage, J.A., Brink, T.L., Rose, T.L., Lum, O., Huang, V., Adey, M., and Leirer, V.O. (1983). Development and validation of a geriatric depression screening scale: A preliminary report. *Journal of Psychiatric Research*, 17, 37-49.

Chapter 5

Counseling and Psychotherapy

There is no question that psychotherapy with older adults is helpful. Studies have shown that psychotherapy with depressed elderly persons is just as effective as with younger adults (Scogin and McElreath, 1994). Even older adults receiving therapy for Major Depression, the most severe type of depression, improve as much as those with milder forms of depression (Scogin and McElreath, 1994). The types of therapy that have been studied and found effective include cognitive, behavioral, interpersonal, reminiscence, and psychodynamic. None of these types of psychotherapy has been proven more effective than the others.

While these results are encouraging, it is more difficult to generalize about how effective psychotherapy is with an LTC population. Two studies using reminiscence therapy found that that it had a positive effect on the mood of LTC residents (Goldwasser, Auerbach, and Harkins, 1987; Rattenbury and Stones, 1989). However, both included a large portion of residents who were not clinically depressed. Thus, their findings cannot necessarily be generalized to LTC residents with significant depression.

Particularly controversial is whether psychotherapy is beneficial for residents with dementia. We believe that therapy can help residents who are not demented or have mild dementia. However, we think that verbal psychotherapy, with the possible exception of Validation Therapy, is unlikely to make a sustained difference in the mood or behavior of moderately to severely demented residents.

We say "verbal psychotherapy" to distinguish it from certain types of therapy that are nonverbal in nature. For example, in Behavior Therapy, interventions are often implemented by the staff or family. Similarly, validation therapy is not just a verbal therapy. The more demented the resident is, the more likely a validating therapist is to use nonverbal techniques (Feil, 1992).

We say that verbal psychotherapy does not make a "sustained difference" because we recognize that even for residents with moderate to severe dementia, any supportive human contact can be valuable, just as visits from family members or the clergy are helpful. Residents are often very lonely and isolated, and their problem behaviors let us know how starved for attention they are.

While verbal psychotherapy may thus comfort a moderately to severely demented resident for the moment, we believe it is usually not cost-effective for Medicare or other insurance to pay for such. Verbal psychotherapy is designed to promote change in behavior and emotional well-being through an ongoing intimate relationship with a therapist. As such, it requires memory for who the therapist is and what was discussed at the last session. Effective psychotherapy has to provide more than momentary companionship for a lonely resident. If such companionship is the most basic need, then staff should attempt to arrange such with the help of family members, the resident's church, peer counseling programs sponsored by community colleges, volunteers, or the family's hiring of a companion for the resident.

One reason that we emphasize this point is that mental health consultants often lose credibility with physicians and other staff when they do verbal psychotherapy with residents who have impaired recent memory and talk incoherently. Once consultants' credibility is lost, it can be difficult to get their support for doing psychotherapy with residents who can benefit from it.

Of course, this all may be a moot point in the future if, as we suspect, Medicare and Medicaid patients are governed by managed care plans. In this situation, psychotherapy will often be denied, even for patients who can benefit from it. In cases where it is authorized, the clinician will probably be limited to just a few sessions.

PSYCHOTHERAPY VERSUS COUNSELING

We believe that social services and nursing staff will have to have basic skills for counseling residents who are emotionally distressed. We say "counseling" because a distinction has traditionally been made between counseling and psychotherapy. Psychotherapy has been viewed as a specialized technique designed to create long-term, beneficial changes in personality, coping, and emotional well-being. Because of its emphasis upon making in-depth changes in the context of an intimate therapeutic relationship, doing psychotherapy has required a professional license. Counseling, by contrast, has been viewed as a more superficial intervention than psychotherapy. Its goals have been viewed as providing empathic support and helping with problems of everyday living. Counseling, the theory goes, is something that anyone with empathy and some basic skills can do.

This definition leads to a picture of "haves" and "have nots." The "haves" are those with professional degrees who know how to do the "real thing" (psychotherapy), whereas the "have nots" are those who can "only" do superficial, concrete counseling. Implicit in this analysis is that psychotherapy is superior to counseling.

We object to this view for two reasons. First, research has compared the effectiveness of professional psychotherapists and that of paraprofessionals, who might be called "counselors." These studies have shown that paraprofessionals are just as effective as the professionals in helping to create behavioral and emotional change (Berman and Norton, 1985). Second, an essential ingredient in any therapy is empathy, the degree to which the therapist is "in tune" with the client. Both psychotherapy and counseling emphasize empathy as the foundation of a therapeutic relationship, and that may be the main reason that both professionals and paraprofessionals are equally effective.

This brings us to our main point: regardless of their academic training, most social services and nursing staff are quite capable of developing empathic relationships with residents and helping them to solve their problems. We do recommend that they pursue some training in counseling that involves some supervised experience and feedback. Courses in peer counseling, for example, are often offered through community colleges and involve some practical experience. Undergraduate courses in psychotherapeutic theory are also helpful.

In this chapter, we provide you with a very brief overview of some basic techniques of psychotherapy that are applicable with LTC residents. We do not believe that simply reading this chapter will make you a good counselor of LTC residents. We provide it as a first step toward helping you to develop rapport with residents and to learn basic counseling techniques. We highly recommend that as you attempt to apply any of these principles, you seek feedback or supervision from a professional, qualified instructor, or experienced peer.

In our overview of these techniques, we discuss their application to depressed residents, because these make up the vast majority of LTC residents who need counseling. However, these approaches can be used with residents who have other problems, such as exaggerated fears or conflicts with other residents.

SUPPORTIVE THERAPY

Supportive therapy is an umbrella term for many counseling activities, but these usually include at least two techniques: empathy and facilitating problem solving. Empathy is the cornerstone of any therapeutic relationship, and it is the chief emphasis in supportive therapy. To provide empathy, a counselor takes every opportunity to convey understanding of the resident's problems and emotions. The counselor often makes reflective comments that mirror the resident's thoughts and feelings. For example, if a resident complains about her slow, painful recovery from a broken hip, the counselor might say, "It sounds as if you're frustrated with your slow recovery—it can get pretty discouraging." While the counselor may ask questions, the emphasis is upon using such empathic reflections to get the resident to explore her own thoughts and feelings about an issue. As such, this approach is often called "nondirective," because the client is allowed to lead the counselor through a process of emotional self-examination.

For depressed residents in LTC, the focus of counseling is often upon helping a resident to face and accept the losses which led to his placement. Empathic counseling can facilitate a resident's grieving and acceptance of these losses. We often notice that residents who at first vociferously protest their LTC placement gradually come to accept it later on. Counseling might speed the process of acceptance by providing a forum in which the resident can describe her grief and frustrations about the placement.

In addition to empathy, supportive therapy usually involves helping the resident to solve his own problems. While staff must sometimes give advice or solve a problem for the resident, the preference in supportive therapy is to help the resident find his own solution. For example, if a resident is having conflict with a roommate over how loud his TV is played, the counselor can ask the resident to think of ways to address this with his roommate. Hopefully, if a resident solves his own problem, this will lead to a greater sense of independence and self-mastery.

REMINISCENCE THERAPY

At first, it may seem strange to think of reminiscing as a type of therapy. After all, if residents are preoccupied with the past, will they not ignore present problems? While this can happen, reminiscing in the elderly can have beneficial consequences for their emotional health. Young people have their entire lives in front of them and thus are rightly occupied with planning for the future. Their focus is upon integrating future goals with what they are doing today. By contrast, LTC residents have most of their lives behind them, and their focus is upon integrating their past with their present. Reminiscing may help residents to answer the question, "What did I do with my life and why?" Reminiscing "is not simply the recounting of historical events, but is instead the unique creation of the individual, representing a dynamically meaningful synthesis of memories which serves to maintain personal identity" (Lesser et al., 1981, p. 295).

In reminiscence therapy, the main technique is to have residents reflect upon the key events of their lives. There are at least three reasons why this may prove emotionally beneficial. First, we hope that this will help residents to "retain emotional and mental contact with a part of themselves that, in the past, was healthier and perhaps more capable of coping" (Sadavoy, 1992, p. 229). As they recall past accomplishments, they may feel the same sense of gratification and empowerment that they did at the time. Second, reminiscence may reduce guilt about past deeds by enabling them to "reinterpret their past actions and feelings," thus leading them to greater "acceptance of the past" (Perrotta and Meacham, 1981, p. 26). Reducing guilt in this way is particularly important for depressed residents, since guilt and self-criticism often accompany depression. Finally, reminiscence therapy can offer a brief, refreshing "retreat from the here and now" (Lesser et al., 1981, p. 292).

A counselor can do reminiscence therapy in either a structured or unstructured way. In unstructured reminiscence, the counselor allows the resident to discuss whatever events from the past he wants. In structured reminiscence, the counselor provides a topic and perhaps a set of follow-up questions. For example, Rattenbury and Stones (1989) had group participants discuss the following topics: childhood and adolescent experiences, work experiences, memories of World War II and the Depression, the impact of TV and other technologies, marriage and children, and later life memories. Fry (1983) also used a structured approach, having clients describe five stressful life events and asking them questions about various dimensions of these events. These dimensions included their feelings at the time, their ways of coping, and any current, unresolved feelings that they had about the events. For LTC residents, it is often desirable to use some degree of structured reminiscence, because they often need cues, such as those above, to stimulate their long-term memory.

While reminiscence therapy can be done on an individual basis, it is ideally suited for groups. The counselor leading a reminiscence group should offer empathic reflections as residents reminisce, and thus model active listening for the group. Often two or more people relate similar experiences and feelings about a topic or phase of life, and the counselor should underscore these commonalities. In this way, she can foster a greater sense of shared experience within the group, which leads to validation of feelings and a sense of group identity.

VALIDATION THERAPY

Fortunately, there is one type of therapy that has been developed specifically for adults with dementia: validation therapy. Created by Naomi Feil, ACSW, validation therapy uses simple techniques with disoriented old-old adults (those 80 years old or more). This therapy is designed to help residents with a wide variety of emotional and behavioral problems, not just depression.

Ms. Feil developed her therapy after finding it frustrating to attempt to orient these residents to present reality. Sensing that each resident is trapped in a "world of fantasy," she "abandoned the goal of reality orientation when I found group members withdrew, or became increasingly hostile, whenever I tried to orient them to an intolerable present reality" (Feil, 1992, p. 9). Instead of orienting them to reality, she "validated" the feelings and needs behind their distorted perceptions by empathizing with them in a multimodal fashion.

What are these feelings and needs of the disoriented old-old that need validation? Feil gives the following answer:

> Alone in an apartment or trapped in a geriatric chair, they return to the time when they were somebody. They use their vivid memories to restore the past, when they were useful, productive, loved. They go back to a time when what they thought and did really counted . . . The old-old express three basic human needs: (1) to be safe and loved; (2) to be useful and productive; (3) to express raw emotions but they no longer express these needs with people in the "here and now;" and (4) their communication is with people and objects from their past. (Feil, 1992, pp. 23-24)

When these needs and emotions are validated, Feil believes that residents experience enhanced self-esteem, increased verbal and nonverbal communication, relief of anxiety and anger, and fewer repetitive behaviors like pacing and pounding (Feil, 1992).

To help residents express these feelings and meet these needs, validating counselors ignore factual errors and misperceptions in order to communicate understanding of the person's subjective world. Therapists use an array of techniques, depending upon a client's level of impairment in cognition and communication. For more intact, expressive clients, the techniques are more verbal, while for the more impaired and less expressive, they are more nonverbal. Verbal techniques include reminiscing; rephrasing "the gist of what the person has said using their key words"; asking concrete factual questions like "what" and "who" rather than insight-oriented questions like "why"; and using "polarity," which is asking for the extreme instance of a given complaint (Feil, 1992, p. 65). To illustrate the use of polarity, Feil gives the following example: "Resident: 'It hurts.' Worker: 'How bad is the pain? When is it the worst?'" (Feil, 1992, p. 65). Asking for the extreme validates the resident's concern by encouraging her to tell the counselor just how bad it is. Nonverbal techniques of validation therapy include using "genuine, direct, prolonged eye contact;" talking in a "clear, low, warm, loving voice tone;" touching in therapeutic ways; matching "their emotion with your face, body, breathing, and voice tone;" and "mirroring" the resident's nonverbal style in order to understand what hisunderlying needs and feelings are (Feil, 1992, pp. 69-70, 74).

The greatest value of validation therapy may lie in its providing a healthy corrective to the traditional emphasis upon Reality Orientation, in which staff constantly correct disoriented residents in order to ground them in present reality. Dietch, Hewett, and Jones (1989) note that Reality Orientation "may attempt to bring unwilling subjects back to an intolerable reality–only to provoke anger, misery, or both" (p. 974). They describe three case examples of residents who had mistaken beliefs about their relatives, such as that deceased relatives were alive or that a son was still a little boy. These residents became angry and agitated when reality orientation was used to correct their mistaken perceptions. However, when validation techniques were used, these residents responded positively. For example, one woman was encouraged to talk about her parents as if they were still alive, which caused her to reminisce about pleasurable times that she had had with them. In another case, a man with Alzheimer's, who thought he saw his deceased brother in the mirror, was encouraged to talk about his brother. As a result, he talked "excitedly and happily about his brother, with whom he was very close," and he could then be "focused on another subject of conversation or activity" (Dietch, Hewett, and Jones, 1989, p. 975).

Concerning research on validation therapy, there is anecdotal evidence like the cases above, and Feil (1992) describes some unpublished research studies. Unfortunately, we do not know of any published controlled studies which have evaluated its effectiveness.

COGNITIVE THERAPY

Cognitive therapy assumes that emotional distress is caused, not as much by stressful events, but by our perceptions of those events.

The theory holds that these cognitive perceptions of events determine whether we feel sad, elated, or indifferent. Seeing the glass as half full or half empty makes all the difference. When it comes to depression, cognitive theory says that depressed people are more likely to perceive what happens to them in distorted ways, which lead them to depressive conclusions about themselves and their world.

As described by Beck et al. (1979), cognitive therapy teaches residents how to combat these highly distorted perceptions that lead to depression. Known as "cognitive distortions," these self-critical perceptions are identified during therapy and then examined to see if there is good evidence to support them. Burns (1980) describes ten cognitive distortions, including "overgeneralization," "magnification," "disqualifying the positive," and "personalizing" (pp. 40-41). In overgeneralizing and magnifying, a depressed resident takes one event and draws a sweeping, pessimistic conclusion from it. In disqualifying the positive, a resident ignores evidence that disconfirms her negative conclusions about herself, such as compliments. In personalizing, the resident sees herself as the cause of an unpleasant event, such as a nurse's speaking to her in an irritable tone of voice, when in fact, she did nothing to cause it. The therapist teaches the resident to identify these implicit perceptions on a daily basis and to challenge them, rather than letting them get her down.

Now let us look at an example of how a depressed resident might use overgeneralizing and magnifying to get himself depressed. A resident who has mild memory problems may become quite distressed over forgetting that he had agreed to play bingo at 3 p.m. yesterday. He may overgeneralize and magnify this event as follows: "This just proves that I can't remember anything anymore. I've lost my mind." Obviously, a resident who interprets it this way is more likely to be depressed than one who sees it the following way: "I'm frustrated that I forgot about bingo yesterday. I know that I don't remember things like I used to, so I'll have to make a point of writing these meetings down." The therapist's task is to help the resident identify the distorted interpretations like the first one, and to help him revise them in favor of the second kind. The hope is that the resident will eventually learn to do this on his own without the therapist's help.

In intervening in a case like this one, the therapist might ask the client a series of questions that helps him to see how distorted his perception is. The purpose of these questions is to help the resident to explore evidence for and against his perception, so that he can revise it in a more realistic, self-affirming direction. Thus, the therapist could ask,"Are there any meetings that you did remember recently?" in order to establish that the resident has recently recalled some appointments. If he replied "no," the therapist might try other ways of demonstrating that the resident can recall some things, such as asking if he can recall yesterday's activity or what was just served for lunch. If the resident demonstrates some recall, the therapist could point this out as evidence against the resident's conclusion that he has no memory.

Obviously, such a technique may only be used on a resident who has no more than mild dementia and is motivated to look into the causes of his depression. In many LTC cases, a purely cognitive approach is not used. Rather, a counselor may use a supportive approach, but remain alert for times that the resident is distorting events. At that time, she can use some of these questions to help the resident to examine the evidence and to revise his interpretation.

BEHAVIOR THERAPY

There are two main types of behavior therapy. One type of behavior therapy is similar to other psychotherapeutic approaches in that client and therapist meet for sessions and work out behavioral strategies for combating depression. These strategies often involve having the client change daily activities so that they give him a sense of pleasure and accomplishment (Beck et al., 1979). This is a very helpful and practical approach for use in LTC. We will cover more specific applications of this model in Chapter 7, where we discuss psychosocial interventions for depression.

Another type of behavior therapy is when behavior is analyzed outside the context of a therapeutic relationship, and interventions are designed for the resident, often without her being told. This approach is most often used with residents who cannot engage in collaborative therapy because of their dementia. We will teach this type of behavior therapy in Chapter 6.

AN INTEGRATED APPROACH

In counseling depressed LTC residents, we believe that using an integrated approach makes most sense. We recommend using a primarily supportive approach with most LTC residents, but one that can be supplemented with other techniques. For example, if a resident likes to reminisce, you could permit the resident to do this while using questioning and reflection to shape her exploration of the past. For disoriented residents who live in the past, you could use validation techniques to affirm the underlying emotion and needs that they are expressing. For residents who distort what happens to them, you could question their misinterpretations using a cognitive approach.

Once again, however, we emphasize that you should only use counseling techniques that you have studied carefully and that you have received some minimal coaching, consultation, or supervision in performing. If you have not had the opportunity for such, we recommend that you use a simple, supportive approach.

GROUP COUNSELING

Any of the above approaches to individual counseling can be applied in group counseling. Lichtenberg (1994) emphasizes that with LTC residents, the primary goals of group therapy should be relieving isolation and promoting interaction, not improving residents' thinking or teaching them skills. These goals are particularly important for our depressed residents, because they are often quite withdrawn.

Before starting a group, you need to make some key decisions about the group. Specific factors that you need to consider include the following:

- What is the focus and purpose of the group?
- Will the group be time-limited or ongoing?
- Will you admit new members to the group after the first week?
- Will you have only cognitively intact residents or a mixture of demented and cognitively intact?
- What counseling techniques will you use?

- How much will you structure the group versus allowing the group to choose its own course?
- How will you get all the residents to the group on time?
- Will you ask the members to agree to confidentiality?

Ideally, you would consult with your mental health consultant about these issues as you design your group. Having your consultant observe your leading a group and providing feedback afterwards would be quite valuable. Of course, if your consultant is available to co-lead a few sessions with you, this would be even more helpful. If you do not have a consultant, hopefully you can find an experienced peer or instructor who can give you advice on these issues and feedback as you plan and conduct the group.

Finally, in LTC groups, there is often not an obvious line between a socialization group and a counseling group. For this reason, you may wish to involve your activities coordinator in designing or leading the group. Reminiscence groups, in particular, may be appealing to the activities coordinator.

CONCLUSION

We have discussed a number of techniques in this chapter, but the most important aspect of counseling is not really a technique: it is empathy. Without empathy, we risk choosing the wrong technique. With empathy, we may not need to use many techniques.

Of course, with many of our demented residents, verbal questioning often does not help us to understand them or what is causing their problem behaviors. For these residents, a behavioral assessment is often necessary, which brings us to our next topic.

REFERENCES

Beck, A.T., Rush, A.J., Shaw, B.F., and Emery, G. (1979). *Cognitive therapy of depression*. New York: Guilford.

Berman, J.S. and Norton, N.C. (1985). Does professional training make a therapist more effective? *Psychological Bulletin, 98*, 401-407.

Burns, D.D. (1980). *Feeling good: The new mood therapy*. New York: William Morrow.

Dietch, J.T., Hewett, L.J., and Jones, S. (1989). Adverse effects of reality orientation. *Journal of the American Geriatric Society*, 37, 974-976.

Feil, N. (1992). *V/F Validation: The Feil Method*. Cleveland: Edward Feil Productions.

Fry, P.S. (1983). Structured and unstructured reminiscence training and depression in the elderly. *Clinical Gerontologist*, 1, 15-37.

Goldwasser, A.N., Auerbach, S.M., and Harkins, S.W. (1987). Cognitive, affective, and behavioral effects of reminiscence group therapy on demented elderly. *International Journal of Aging and Human Development*, 25, 209-222.

Lesser, J., Lazarus, L.W., Frankel, R., and Havasy, S. (1981). Reminiscence group therapy with psychotic geriatric inpatients. *The Gerontologist*, 21, 291-296.

Lichtenberg, P. (1994). *A guide to psychological practice in geriatric long-term care*. Binghamton, New York: The Haworth Press.

Perrotta, P. and Meacham, J.A. (1981). Can a reminiscing intervention alter depression and self-esteem? *International Journal of Aging and Human Development*, 14, 23-30.

Rattenbury, C. and Stones, M.J. (1989). A controlled evaluation of reminiscence and current topics discussion groups in a nursing home context. *Gerontologist*, 29, 768-771.

Sadavoy, J. (1992). Psychotherapy for the institutionalized elderly. In D.K. Conn, N. Herrmann, A. Kaye, D. Rewilak, A. Robinson, and B. Schogt (Eds.), *Practical psychiatry in the nursing home* (pp. 217-236). Seattle: Hogrefe and Huber.

Scogin, F. and McElreath, L. (1994). Efficacy of psychosocial treatments for geriatric depression: A quantitative review. *Journal of Consulting and Clinical Psychology*, 1, 69-74.

Chapter 6

Designing Behavioral Assessments and Interventions

One of the most challenging aspects of working in LTC is the behavioral problems that we must address. In the last chapter, we talked about how counseling might help a resident to address emotional problems. In Chapter 7, we make specific suggestions for dealing with certain behavioral problems. In this chapter, we teach you how to do a behavioral analysis of the problem, so that you leave no stone unturned in trying to figure out why a resident is behaving in a certain way. Your behavioral analysis can, in turn, lead to very specific interventions for that resident's problem.

THE ABCs OF BEHAVIOR

In order to analyze the causes of behavioral problems, we have to look at what comes before and after the behavior. An easy way to describe this chain of events is to label its links as "A," "B," and "C," which are defined in Table 6.1. A *Behavior* ("B") is preceded by one or more *Activators* events ("A"), which serve as a trigger for the behavior. These antecedent events (activators) function as an alarm bell that lets the person know that there is an opportunity to meet a need or to obtain a certain goal. The *Consequences* ("C") following the behavior determine whether the person is more or less likely to repeat the behavior in the future. In describing the consequences, we often say that the behavior was "reinforced" or "not reinforced," depending upon whether or not the person received satisfying consequences from the behavior.

TABLE 6.1.The ABCs of Behavior

- Activator: what precedes the behavior; the trigger.
- Behavior: what the person does.
- Consequences: the reinforcing results of the behavior.

Here is a simple example of this behavioral chain that might apply to us:

Activator: Feeling hungry and stressed-out after a hard day at work, you are standing in the supermarket check-out line.

Behavior: You add two candy bars to your purchases and eat them on the way home.

Consequence: You feel less hungry and calmer.

Here, feeling hungry and stressed-out while standing next to candy bars ("A") was a trigger for the behavior ("B") of purchasing and eating two candy bars. The consequences ("C") were that you were reinforced through pleasure and physical and emotional relief. Some of you might say, "But what about the guilt I'd feel afterwards?" That would likely come after you had eaten the candy bars and already received the pleasurable rewards. As we mention below, the consequences which immediately follow the behavior are the most powerful ones.

How does knowing the ABCs help us to change behavior? Once we have identified the activators of the behavior, we can attempt to eliminate these triggers wherever possible, and perhaps provide different activators that will lead to desired behavior. Once we have identified the reinforcing consequences, we can help staff change how they respond to the person, so that they reinforce desired behavior instead of the problematic behavior.

Returning to the example above, if you wanted to make it less likely that you would impulsively buy and eat two candy bars, you would change the chain of activators and/or consequences. In this case you could change the activators by shopping for food when you are *not* hungry and stressed-out. If you do shop when hungry and stressed-out, you could buy a healthier food before getting to the check-out line, where the candy bars would tempt you, and then could eat the healthier food on the way home. In this case, you would experience the reinforcing consequences of pleasure and relief for a different behavior: eating a healthier food.

Keep in mind that consequences which appear negative may still be reinforcing. The best example is the patient who cries out repeatedly, only to receive harsh feedback, such as "Shut up!" from other patients. Such feedback may still be reinforcing, in that the resident does receive attention and a response from the environment which alone may be somewhat satisfying. For some people, negative attention is better than none at all.

TYPES OF ACTIVATORS

Cohn, Smyer, and Horgas (1991) describe two types of activators: internal and external. Internal activators are "human needs that drive us to act," whereas external activators are "physical features of the environment and what goes on around us" (p. 17). Internal activators can be physical or emotional in nature, and external activators can be environmental or social in nature. Some examples of these are listed in Table 6.2.

TABLE 6.2. Types of Activators

Internal Activators

- *Physical:* hunger/thirst, too warm/cold, pain, need to eliminate.
- *Mental/emotional:* sadness, anxiety, loneliness, fatigue, frustration, need for stimulation, delirium, hallucinations, delusions.

External Activators

- *Environmental:* noises, barriers, wheelchair collisions.
- *Social:* caregiving by staff, demands or requests from staff, presence of certain residents or staff members, sudden movements by others, yelling by another resident, conflict with roommate.

To return to our personal example above, the internal activators for buying the candy bars were both physical (hunger) and emotional (stressed-out). The external activators were social (having to stand in a line of people) and environmental (standing next to candy bars).

IDENTIFYING ACTIVATORS AND CONSEQUENCES

To identify activators and consequences, you need to put on your detective hat and ask key questions, which are summarized in Table 6.3. These are questions that any detective would ask when building a good case, or that any journalist would ask when writing a good story. An easy way to remember them is that five of the six questions begin with the letter "w": the *who, what, when, where, why,* and *how* of the behavior.

In asking the *when, where,* and *why* questions, we are looking for clues to internal and external activators. In asking the *who, what,* and *how* questions, we are looking for all parts of the behavioral chain: activators, behavior, and consequences.

TABLE 6.3. Playing Sherlock Holmes: Key Questions for Identifying Activators and Consequences

- *What* is the behavior, and what happens before and after?
- *Who* are the people involved?
- *When* does it occur?
- *Where* does it occur?
- *Why* does the behavior occur (e.g., internal activators)?
- *How* do the staff and other residents respond to the behavior?
- *How* does the resident respond, in turn, to their responses?

Now let's look at how we would use these questions to analyze a simple behavioral sequence that could occur in LTC. Consider the following case example:

Jane is sitting in a geri-chair in the hallway. As the nurse scurries past her down the hall, she calls out softly, "Nurse," because she needs toileting. The nurse ignores her because she is preoccupied with other duties. The resident repeats "nurse" in a calm voice, but is again ignored. She begins to call out more and more loudly until she is yelling and pounding on the table. The nurse then asks what she wants and takes her to the bathroom. She is then calm. (Adapted from Cohn, Smyer, and Horgas, 1991, p. 19.)

Now let's ask our detective questions:

- *What* is the problem behavior? Resident's yelling and pounding her fist
- *Who* is involved? Jane and the nursing staff
- *When* does it occur? It occurs when staff are busy and do not respond to her quiet requests.
- *Where* does it occur? In the hallway
- *How* does it occur? Nurse responded only after resident screamed and pounded; resident stopped after receiving attention and toileting.
- *Why* does it occur? Resident needed to use bathroom and feels frustrated when she is ignored.

Notice that these answers flesh out the A-B-C chain for us. The external activators (A) include the hallway and staff's not responding to the resident's quiet requests. The internal activators are the resident's need for toileting and frustration at getting no response. The problem behavior (B) is the resident's screaming and pounding her fist. The consequences (C) are that the nurse provided attention and toileting immediately after the resident screamed and pounded.

By providing attention and toileting immediately after Jane screamed and pounded, the nurse taught her that this is an effective way to get what she needs. In other words, the nurse "reinforced" pounding and screaming and ignored the desired behavior of making quiet requests.

Teaching goes both ways, however. The resident has also influenced how staff will behave toward her in the future. For example, staff could learn from this incident and resolve to respond to Jane's quiet demands in the future, knowing that such may forestall an outburst.

On the other hand, staff could feel angry with Jane, perceiving her as a manipulative, demanding resident who is constantly seeking attention. Staff might show their inner feelings in the future by ignoring her, giving her less attention during care, or speaking curtly with her. Such responses might serve as more triggers for angry outbursts.

This cycle is illustrated in Figures 6.1 and 6.2, which are similar to those portrayed by Ogland-Hand and Florsheim (1994). Notice how the consequences of the problem behavior can be separated into immediate and long-term ones. The immediate consequence is that staff have given the resident attention and toileting. The long-term consequences are staff's actions caused by their emotional response to the resident's outburst: namely, that staff ignore her, give her less attention, and speak curtly to her. These long-term "Cs", in turn, become potential "As" for future outbursts.

Cohn, Smyer, and Horgas (1991) call this two-way learning process "circular learning," in which "people both learn from and teach each other how to behave. The staff teach residents how to behave in certain situations, and the residents teach caregivers how to respond to them" (p. 20).

FIGURE 6.1. The Cycle of Resident-Staff Behavior

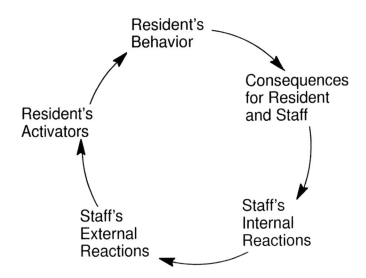

FIGURE 6.2. Example of the Cycle of Resident-Staff Behavior

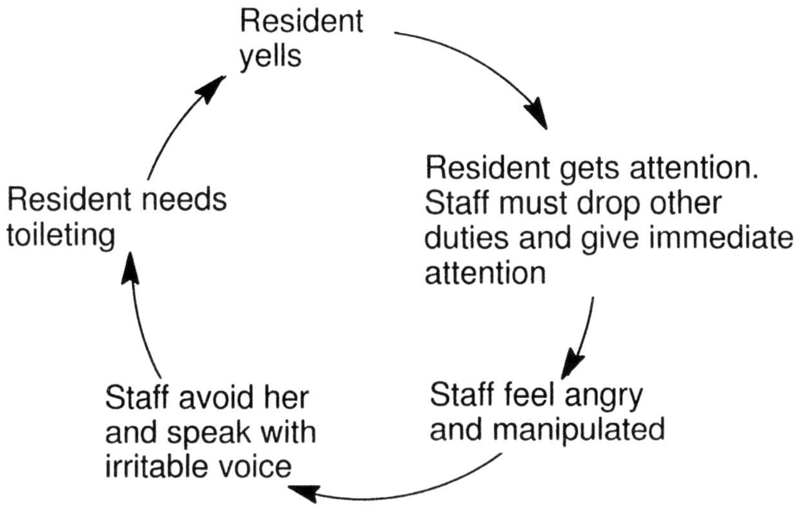

Notice how this cycle expands the A-B-C model to a series of A-B-C chains. The "C" at the end of one chain, such as staff's ignoring or talking irritably to a resident, can become one of the "As" for the next chain. The cycle also expands the simple A-B-C model by including staff's internal emotional reactions to a resident. If these are not acknowledged and dealt with by staff, their negative feelings toward the resident can undermine a good behavioral program.

A TRACKING GRID FOR ASSESSING BEHAVIORAL PROBLEMS

When you are attempting to identify the activators and conse-quences of a behavior, asking staff for their casual observations of the problem is often not enough. Their reports may be contradictory, or staff may selectively remember certain details of the As and Cs while forgetting other very important dimensions. While hashmark tracking is better than nothing, it simply gives the frequency of the behavior and on what shift it occurred, which provides little qualitative information. To avoid these problems, having staff describe the A-B-C chain using a tracking grid is often helpful. A tracking grid is a table with a series of columns asking staff to record the *who, what, when*, and *where* of the problem behavior.

Examples of such a grid are shown in Figures 6.3 and 6.4. In the first example, Ms. D's screaming, the "Time" and "Place" columns give us clues to external activators. Because it is a behavior that is often prolonged, the length of time that she screamed is included, which gives us a sense of how severe the incident was and how quickly staff brought it under control. Under the "Cause" column, staff were asked to pinpoint the reason for the screaming if they could. Such would provide more information about internal and external activators. The "Staff's Response" column tells us what the consequences were for her screaming. The "Result" column tells us how successful this response was in addressing the behavior.

In the second example, Mr. L's Hitting and Wandering (Figure 6.4), staff were concerned about two behavioral problems and thus both were tracked simultaneously. This grid is similar to the first except that staff must designate the "Type of Behavior," whether it is hitting or wandering. There is no column for the "Length" of time the behavior occurred, because hitting and wandering are not usually protracted behaviors.

If you wish to avoid creating a tracking grid for each individual resident, you could design a generic one for use with most residents. Such a grid is shown in Figure 6.5.

Tips on Implementing a Tracking Grid

Even the best tracking grid will prove worthless if the staff are not motivated to use it. Consequently, we strongly recommend that before having staff track the behavior, you get a consensus from the staff that the behavior is serious enough to invest time in tracking. Otherwise, since it requires extra work, they may not cooperate.

Once they have agreed, you can give staff a grid and have them track the residents' behavior using the grid for a week, two weeks, or longer, depending on the behavior's frequency. For a behavior that occurs often, such as calling out, two or three days may provide sufficient data, whereas less frequent behaviors, such as physical aggression, may require a few weeks of tracking.

FIGURE 6.3. Tracking Grid for Ms. D's Screaming

Date	Time	Place	Length (minutes)	Cause (if known)	Staff's Response	Her Response
4-19	5:10 a.m.	Bed	2-3 mins.	Wants to go to BR	Assisted to toilet	Back to bed and quiet
4-19	9:15 a.m.	Room	5 mins.	(was talking Italian) BR but refused	Asked if wanted to go	Quiet
4-20	2:00 p.m.	Room	2 mins.	Wants to go to BR	Assisted to toilet	Quiet
4-21	3:25 a.m.	Bed	135 mins.	Talking in Italian, yelling, laughing at the wall, screaming because she thought she was in her kitchen and someone was at the window	Talked with her briefly, then gave IM Haldol	None
4-30	9:00 a.m.	Wheelchair	3-5 mins.	Wants to go to BR	Assisted to toilet	Quiet

95

FIGURE 6.4. Tracking Grid for Mr. L's Hitting and Wandering

Date	Time	Place	Type of Behavior (hitting, wandering)	What Staff Did (if known)	His Response	Comments
8-29	6:00 p.m.	Other residents' rooms: 2 and 46	Wandering	Approached calmly and offered to take him back to room	Spoke foul language	
8-31	6:30 p.m.	Wandering room to room and inside and outside facility	Combative, wandering, yelling	Called 911, approached calmly	Calmed down only when police came	
9-1	1:00 p.m.	Room 18 (not his)	Wandering	Redirected	No resistance	
9-2	1:25 p.m.	DSD Office	Combative after wandered there	Tried to take him away from office	Verbally abusive, tried to hit CNA	Talked with him calmly
9-2	2:00 p.m.	Room 17 (not his)	Combative after wandered there	Tried to take him out of the room	Verbally abusive, tried to hit CNA	Talked with him calmly
9-3	2:00 p.m.	Room 33 (not his)	Combative after wandered there	Redirection given	Verbally abusive, tried to hit CNA	Talked with him calmly
9-9	2:30 p.m.	Outside facility by the door	Combative and yelling after wandering outside	Calmly explained to him why he has to go inside	Resistant for a while, but quiet after 5 mins.	

FIGURE 6.5. Generic Behavioral Tracking Grid

Resident: _____   Problem Behavior(s): _____

Date	Time	Place	Behavior	Cause (if known)	Staff's Response	Resident's Response	Comments

You should not be surprised if tracking the behavior in this way appears to reduce its frequency. Sometimes staff's observing the behavior closely provides the patient with more attention, which by itself may reduce the problem behavior. Staff may also monitor their own behavior more closely, which may cause them to change the way that they respond to the person. Another explanation for low frequency is that the behavior may simply not be occurring as often as staff think.

CHANGING BEHAVIOR BY CHANGING ACTIVATORS AND CONSEQUENCES

Cohn, Smyer, and Horgas (1991) describe a simple formula for changing behavior: eliminating old activators and reinforcers (consequences) for undesired behavior, and substituting new activators and reinforcers for desired behavior. To illustrate using our last case example, we would want to eliminate the old activator of the nurse's not responding to the resident when the resident softly asked to go to the bathroom. We would want the nurse to reinforce the quiet request by providing immediate help thereafter (a new consequence). Even if the nurse were too busy to provide immediate toileting, she could still acknowledge the request and let the resident know that she would be there soon, thus providing immediate attention (another new consequence). If in the future the resident again yelled and pounded, we would want the nurse to respond with as little attention as possible in taking her to the bathroom, so that reinforcement of the behavior was minimized (a revised consequence).

Keep in mind that often changing the activators alone may be enough to change the problem behavior. In our example above, scheduling regular toileting intervals for the resident (e.g., every two hours) might prevent her from needing toileting during the nurses' busiest periods. Examples of ways to change internal and external activators are presented in Table 6.4.

When attempting to change the consequences of behavior in an LTC setting, *social reinforcement* is the simplest approach. Social reinforcement means providing attention, touch, help, eye contact,

TABLE 6.4. Ways to Eliminate Internal or External Activators

Internal Activator	One Suggestion for Eliminating It
• Boredom	Get resident a TV, radio, music box
• Poor vision/hearing	Get resident glasses and hearing aid
• Pain	Address physical causes
• Psychosis	Psychiatric medication

External Activator	One Suggestion for Eliminating It
• Certain time of day	Schedule family visits or activities then
• Wheelchair collisions	Redesign areas where they occur
• Roommate conflict	Change roommates
• Combative during caregiving	Use two CNAs instead of one to start caregiving

or praise after a desired behavior occurs. Social reinforcement is most powerful when it is done *immediately* after the desired behavior. Referring to our previous example, staff could have socially reinforced Jane's quiet requests by responding verbally, giving eye contact, touching her arm, or praising her for asking appropriately.

While there are other types of reinforcers, such as primary reinforcers (e.g., food) or secondary reinforcers (e.g., tokens), administering these involves much more staff time and training. Given staff's many demands, only the simplest intervention is likely to be carried out consistently.

Consistency is one of the most important principles of behavioral intervention. As much as possible, old activators and consequences must be consistently avoided, and the new ones consistently used. One reason that consistency is so important is that when problem behaviors are only occasionally reinforced, they can become even more resistant to change. Of course, maintaining consistency across three shifts, including weekends, is quite challenging in a LTC context.

CASE STUDIES
OF BEHAVIORAL ASSESSMENT

Now we look at two case studies that illustrate how to analyze staff's written content on the tracking grid so that you can arrive at the most accurate conclusions. To do so, we return to the previous tracking grids (Figures 6.3 and 6.4) to find out what the nursing staff actually recorded on these forms.

The results for "Ms. D's screaming" are shown in Figure 6.3. Ms. D was an Italian-American lady who spoke fluent English but, because of her moderate dementia, often returned to speaking Italian. First, we look at the "Date" and "Time" columns to see if the screaming was clustered in one or two days or whether the behavior tended to occur at a particular time of day. The answer to both of these questions is no, although two instances occurred at about 9 a.m. Next, we look at the "Place" column to see if she screamed at a particular place. Four incidents occurred in her room and the fifth is unspecified. The "Length" of the screaming was two to five minutes in four of the cases, but 135 minutes in one case. This prompts us to look at the "Cause" column to see what happened during the short episodes, as compared with the long one. During the long outburst, she was acutely delusional and hallucinating, suggesting that she was experiencing delirium. Her PRN Haldol was then given and she eventually quieted down. By contrast, the four brief episodes had nothing to do with delirium. Three were caused by her wanting to go to the bathroom. As a result of this analysis, staff were advised to offer to take her to the bathroom more often and to do so when she was not screaming. Staff decided to implement a toileting program in which she was taken to the bathroom at regular intervals. After staff implemented this program, she screamed only three times over the next 3.5 weeks–about a 50 percent reduction in her frequency of screaming.

Now let's look at the second case: Mr. L's hitting and wandering (Figure 6.4). Mr. L was fully ambulatory but had severe dementia from advanced Alzheimer's disease. Looking first at the "Date" and "Time" columns, we find that all of the behaviors occurred between 1:00 p.m. and 6:30 p.m. Within that time frame, they were concentrated between 1:00 p.m. and 2:30 p.m. and between 6:00 p.m. and

6:30 p.m.–right after lunch and dinner. While the staff had initially described his hitting and wandering as two separate problems, it is obvious from the "Type of Behavior" column that the two are connected, because he became combative only after wandering somewhere and being confronted by staff. In all cases, staff attempted to redirect him from the area into which he had wandered. In one instance, he cooperated; in another he swore, and in the remaining five, he became combative. One episode was so severe enough that staff called "911." The two main conclusions drawn from this analysis were that (1) he only hits staff after wandering and being confronted, and (2) he only wanders after lunch and dinner.

The key to preventing his hitting, then, was to stop him from wandering after lunch and after dinner. After discussing these results, the Director of Nursing (DON) decided to have him moved from the first meal shift to the second, so that staff could give him attention immediately after lunch and dinner. The DON believed that he might be wandering after meals in search of the bathroom, especially since he had occasionally defecated in the hallway. Thus, she decided that staff would take him to the bathroom immediately after meals. The consultant also suggested that after toileting, they could also escort him on a walk around the patio, so that some of his restless energy could be worked off.

In analyzing the results of these tracking grids, it is often helpful to identify the general behavior patterns and then present them at the care planning meeting. In this way, further observations and inferences, such as those of the DON above, can be considered prior to the formulation of a comprehensive plan.

IS THE INTERVENTION WORKING?

To determine whether a behavioral intervention is working, some kind of quantitative measure is needed. Ideally, the tracking grid used prior to the intervention would be continued, which would provide more qualitative information about how the resident is responding to the new approach. However, given staff's large burden of paperwork, they often prefer to return to simple hashmark tracking after using the grid to get baseline information. While this is not ideal, it still tells you whether the behavior's frequency is changing in the desired direction.

How long should you wait for behavior to change? It often depends upon the frequency of the behavior. If it occurs quite frequently (e.g., a few times a day) during the assessment phase, you should see a change within a few days. For less frequent behaviors, you may need to wait a couple of weeks or more to see if it is working.

Where there is improvement, the problem behavior usually decreases but does not disappear completely. At that point, you can decide whether the reduced frequency is acceptable to staff or not. If not, additional interventions could be considered or the current one could be tried for a longer time.

Sometimes the frequency of the behavior does not decrease much, but the intensity and length of the behavior does. For example, the resident may yell as often but not as loudly or as long as before. Such improvement can still make a big difference in the ability of staff and resident to tolerate the behavior. If staff are only using hashmark tracking during the intervention phase, however, you may not find out that the intensity and length have decreased. In that case, you may only find out about this type of improvement by talking with the nursing staff who work with the resident.

WHEN THE INTERVENTION FAILS

If your first intervention fails, don't be discouraged. Behavioral interventions don't always work, even when well-designed.

When the first one fails, you can discuss alternative behavioral interventions in your multidisciplinary care planning meetings. You can ask staff to think of other triggers or reinforcing consequences that were not considered after the initial assessment. Then you can decide on a new behavioral approach, or you can decide that a combination of behavioral interventions and psychiatric medication should be tried. Alternatively, you may decide that the triggers are internal and thus demand mainly medical interventions or psychiatric medication.

CONCLUSION

Human behavior is complex. In this chapter, we have attempted to cut through this complexity by recommending a simple tracking grid to identify the key causes of problem behavior. Using this grid will help you to arrive at interventions that are simple, but not simplistic. In the next chapter, we hope to expand your repertoire of simple interventions by addressing specific psychosocial and behavioral problems.

REFERENCES

Cohn, M.D., Smyer, M.A., and Horgas, A.L. (1991). *The ABCs of behavior change, skills for working with behavior problems in nursing homes: A guide for trainers* (Workshop Version). University Park, PA: Gerontology Center, Penn State University.

Ogland-Hand, S.M. and Florsheim, M. (1994). *Family work in nursing homes.* Paper presented at the Annual Meeting of the American Psychological Association, Los Angeles.

Chapter 7

Interventions for Specific Psychosocial and Behavioral Problems

Once you have assessed a resident's behavioral or emotional problem(s), you are finally ready to design an intervention. As we discussed in the last chapter, your behavioral analysis of the activators and consequences may lead you to effective interventions. In some cases, however, you may want additional ideas, some of which are provided in this chapter. In addition, there are times when intervention must begin immediately, either because of the behavior's severity or because staff doubt that using the tracking grid would provide insight. In these cases, the interventions below provide a starting point.

We begin with interventions for psychotic residents, because 25 to 50 percent of demented LTC residents display psychotic symptoms (Curlik, Frazier, and Katz, 1991). We then discuss agitated residents, including those who are physically aggressive, who make noise, who verbally abuse others, and who wander. Next, we tackle the sensitive and controversial issue of sexuality in LTC. Finally, we describe psychosocial ways of intervening with depressed residents.

RESPONDING TO DELUSIONAL RESIDENTS

In Chapter 3, we defined paranoid delusions as a false inference about a factual event. The most common type of delusion in LTC is the persecutory type, in which a resident may believe that others are trying to harm her or conspire against her. Here, the *factual event* is that other residents live around her, but the *false inference* is that they are trying to harm her or conspire against her. Other examples of persecutory delusions are a resident's belief that the staff are deliberately abusing her, that her food is poisoned, or that family members are stealing her money. Hallucinations may or may not accompany these delusions.

In LTC, it is important to distinguish such delusions from delusions that are caused by poor memory. Delusions stemming from poor memory can be called "secondary delusions," because they are caused by poor recent memory, not a tendency to misinterpret events (Birkett, 1991, p. 63). The most common type of secondary delusion is a resident's claim that others are stealing from him, when in fact, he had merely forgotten where he had put something.

Causes of Delusions

While schizophrenia can cause delusions, the two most common causes of delusions in LTC are perceptual impairment and cognitive impairment, which often coexist. Concerning perceptual impairment, elderly paranoid patients are more likely to display hearing and visual impairment (Koenig et al., 1996). Hearing impairment may cause a resident to "conclude that others are talking about him," or to "refer to himself fragments of speech that are partially heard" (Christison, Christison, and Blazer, 1989, p. 409). Visually impaired residents may be more likely to misinterpret what staff and others are doing.

However, the major cause of delusions in the elderly is cognitive impairment caused by delirium or dementia (Christison, Christison, and Blazer, 1989). In Chapter 3, we discussed how acute medical problems can quickly cause a mentally normal resident to develop delirium accompanied by delusions. The role of dementia in the development of delusions is not completely understood. From a physical standpoint, the changes in brain structure that accompany dementia may lead to biochemical imbalances that make the person vulnerable to developing psychotic symptoms. In addition, the poor memory and reasoning ability that accompany dementia probably play a role in the development of delusions. Without good memory and reasoning ability, a person is more likely to seize upon one or two pieces of information, which leads her to a distorted interpretation of what is happening.

Case Study 1

To illustrate how a delusion may unfold in an LTC resident, we briefly summarize a case presented by Carstenson and Fremouw (1981). These authors describe a delusional 68-year-old woman, Ms. B, who was confined to a wheelchair and refused to wear a hearing aid for her moderate hearing loss. She was bothered at having lost her "individuality and independence" after entering the home, and thus "found it aversive to request any kind of assistance from the staff" (p. 330). While living at a previous nursing home the year before, Ms. B had complained of abuse by two male aides, and the authors thought that this probably had occurred. Upon arriving at her present nursing home, she claimed that a male aide, whom she had known at a previous nursing home, was trying to kill her with "a deer rifle, Tylenol (to which she was allergic), or poisoning with lye" (p. 330). Over a period of several weeks, she became more and more anxious about being killed and began to suspect more people of wanting to harm her. Ms. B reported that her hearing ability vacillated, but when she could hear, she heard "threats from her alleged murderer" (p. 330). The staff's response to her allegations "included avoidance, confrontation, reassurance, and, according to Ms. B, sometimes agreement" (p. 331).

Carstenson and Fremouw (1981) offer an explanation for the development of this delusion. First, they point out that a delusion often has its roots in a real event or threat that the person faced at some point. In Ms. B's case, this was the reported physical abuse by the two male aides. Another stressor for her was her disabilities, which left her confined to a wheelchair and hearing impaired, both of which served to keep her more isolated from staff. Without the hearing ability to "receive corrective feedback, the likelihood of mistaken interpretations was increased" (p. 331). Consequently, faced with the "ambiguous and often contradictory information" from her everyday life, she was predisposed to explain the information by "the acceptance of a false belief" (p. 331). This false belief caused her to further isolate herself from the threatening community. The resulting isolation provided her with few opportunities to find evidence that staff were not a threat to her. Her delusion was also maintained by the occasional validation of her fears that she received from staff and her family.

Intervening with the Delusional Resident

In intervening with a delusional resident, the most important principle is that we do not argue or challenge the delusion when the resident describes it. Arguing against it can sometimes strengthen the person's conviction about his delusion, because he often redoubles his effort to convince us that he is right. The more he argues for his delusion, the more he looks for confirming evidence, and the more entrenched the delusion becomes.

If we cannot argue against it, what should we do? Carstenson and Fremouw (1981) recommend ignoring delusional statements and reinforcing nondelusional statements. With Ms. B, the resident described above, the authors instructed the staff to respond as follows:

> Whenever Ms. B spoke of her fears, the staff was instructed to say that they understood that someone was coming to talk to her about her concerns and to immediately direct the conversation to another topic. They were also asked to initiate conversations with Ms. B at times when she was not verbalizing her concerns, so that conversations would not be limited to those initiated by paranoid statements. (p. 331)

When using this approach, you should advise family members to do the same when they visit. Family members often are at a loss as to how to respond to their relative's delusion and often welcome such guidance. In cases where the resident believes that family members are persecuting her and is hostile toward them, you can suggest that they take a break from visitation for a few days. Family members are often relieved at this suggestion, because they find it exasperating and frustrating to visit an accusing relative.

In some instances, a resident is so obsessed with his delusion that he insists upon getting feedback about it. Here, staff can empathize with the resident's distress without agreeing with the mistaken belief. For example, a staff member could say: "I understand how you see things. I don't share your view, but I do understand how frightened you are."

Antipsychotic medication is often given to a resident who has delusions, particularly when the delusion is accompanied by hallucinations, distresses the resident a great deal, and/or leads to disruption in activities of daily living (ADLs). Such medication often calms the resident, but does not dissolve the delusion. In such cases, you still need to apply the above approach so that the resident's delusional thinking may be minimized.

Case Illustration

Ms. O, an 85-year-old woman, was admitted from the acute hospital following coronary bypass surgery and had diagnoses of cerebrovascular disease and diabetes. A former librarian, she had never married and had no living relatives. She exhibited moderate dementia with poor hearing and vision. She was not taking psychiatric medication.

Ms. O had a delusion that men were hiding in her closet at night so that they could rape her. She was obsessed with paying her bill and thus frequently asked staff how much she owed the home and how much was left in her bank account.

The facility had a Psychotropic Medication Committee (see Chapter 8), which recommended a low dose of Haldol. Staff were instructed to avoid arguing with her, to identify triggers for her talking about her delusion, and, once she began talking about her delusion, to divert her to another topic. They also were instructed to avoid whispering or speaking in low tones when she was nearby, so that she could hear what staff were saying. To show her that there was no evidence for her delusion, her closet was inspected periodically by the administrator and the maintenance staff. To address her obsession with paying her bills, the administrator created a "bill for services" on the facility's letterhead, on which he stamped "paid in full." Staff put this in her bedside drawer so that when she asked about her bill, they could show it to her. Finally, given her background as a librarian, the activities director obtained a moveable rack and filled it with donated books and magazines, which occupied her time and gave her a sense of purpose. Within three months, her delusions ceased and she expressed less frequent concern about her bill. At that point, the Psychotropic Medication Committee could discuss the possibility of recommending that her Haldol be decreased or discontinued.

RESIDENTS WHO HALLUCINATE

As you may recall from Chapter 3, a hallucination is a perception without a stimulus, and the most common types are visual and auditory. Hallucinations differ from illusions, which anyone can experience from time to time. Illusions occur when "an actual external stimulus is misperceived or misinterpreted" (APA, 1994, p. 767).

As with delusions, elderly people with hearing and visual problems are at greater risk for developing hallucinations (Christison, Christison, and Blazer, 1989). Recall that in the case of Ms. B, the hearing-impaired resident described above, her delusion of persecution was accompanied by her hearing the voice of her alleged assailant.

We should emphasize that hallucinations are not always abnormal. Recently bereaved people often experience hallucinations as a normal part of the grieving process. During the weeks and months following the death of a spouse or other family member, they may experience visual and auditory hallucinations of the deceased person. They may also search for the relative, have a sense that he is with them, or talk to him (Shuchter and Zisook, 1993). In the case of grieving residents, staff should not perceive these symptoms as problematic. In fact, grieving residents may be frightened by these symptoms and may need staff's reassurance that they are normal.

Medication

Antipsychotic medication, including Haldol and Risperdal, is the most common intervention for hallucinations. However, as with delusions, medication often mutes hallucinations without causing them to disappear. For example, a medicated person may report that he still hears voices but that they are less intrusive, less loud, or less frequent. For this reason, psychosocial interventions are still important in intervening with hallucinating residents.

Another reason is that not all hallucinating residents need antipsychotic medication. Some hallucinate only occasionally. Others do so often, but are not distressed by the hallucinations, or are not so preoc-cupied that their daily activities are disrupted. For others, it is difficult to tell if the person is experiencing hallucinations or merely illusions. In these cases, the attending physician may not want to prescribe medication unless the hallucinations worsen.

Psychosocial Interventions

Hallucinating residents are very prone to misinterpreting what is going on around them. For this reason, Hussian (1986) recommends approaching these residents in a way which minimizes "the likelihood that visual and auditory information will be misinterpreted by the client" (p. 133). Specifically, he recommends that staff "move slowly into the visual field of these clients," and that they "interact from the front of the client and move slowly" (p. 133). Similarly, preventing other residents from wandering into the person's room is important, because the hallucinating resident may become alarmed about what they are doing (Hussian, 1986).

Another way to prevent hallucinating patients from misinterpreting events is through environmental intervention. If a room is dimly lit, a resident is more likely to misinterpret what is going on in the shadows. For this reason, increasing the lighting may prevent an illusion or hallucination, provided that it does not increase glare. Predictability of environment is also important, and thus Robinson, Spencer, and White (1989) recommend changing it as little as possible. If a room change is necessary, they recommend having "a trusted caregiver explain the new environment" (p. B-3). Finally, since visual and auditory impairment are often present in those who hallucinate, staff should make sure that their hearing and vision are corrected as much as possible.

Case Study

Mr. M, a 74-year-old Hispanic resident with moderate Alzheimer's dementia, was referred for psychological evaluation because of frightening auditory hallucinations. He had been taking Haldol for psychosis for several months, and his symptoms had been in remission. However, once he contracted a urinary tract infection, his psychotic symptoms returned with a vengeance. When his relatives visited, he told them that he had heard voices threatening to take him from the home; break his legs, toes, nose, and glasses; steal his watch; and pull out his teeth. He complained about having nightmares of this happening to him. At one point, he thought he had overheard a staff member telling someone that they would remove him from the nursing home that night.

As the Haldol was continued and his urinary tract infection cleared up, the intensity of his hallucinations diminished greatly over the next two weeks. He still believed that someone would "kick" him out of the nursing home, but did not express fear of any physical abuse.

Over the next year, Mr. M displayed few signs of psychosis and thus, nursing staff asked his physician to discontinue the Haldol. While he did well for several months thereafter, he eventually became psychotic again. During this episode, he reported the delusions that he had a disease manifested by a rash on his back, that staff might take away his clothes, that his room was bugged, and that someone was looking in the window at him. He heard derogatory voices "telling me I am a thief and good for nothing." He said the man behind the voice was "John," who "knows everything I'm doing."

At this point, he was referred for another psychological evaluation. The cognitive screening showed that over the last 18 months, his cognitive impairment had progressed from moderate to severe. Nursing staff discussed psychiatric medication with the physician, who reinstituted the Haldol. Over the next few months, the intensity and frequency of his delusions and hallucinations decreased, but he still occasionally heard voices.

This case illustrates the fluctuating course and multiple causes of hallucinations and delusions. While his initial psychosis was probably caused by his Alzheimer's dementia, the sudden return of florid symptoms may have been caused by his urinary tract infection. Fortunately, this episode passed and staff were able to take him off the Haldol for several months. However, his psychotic symptoms eventually returned in full force. The reason for this second episode is not clear, but his continuing cognitive deterioration may have contributed.

Ruling Out Medical Causes of Psychosis

We end this section with a reminder that, as discussed in Chapter 3, hallucinations and delusions often accompany delirium. Since delirium is always caused by illnesses or medications, ruling out delirium is very important in assessing a resident's psychosis. Where staff establish that delirium is the cause of psychotic symptoms, treating its medical causes will eventually relieve these symptoms.

AGITATION

Agitation is an umbrella term for many disruptive behaviors. Agitation can be defined as "inappropriate verbal, vocal, or motor activity" (Cohen-Mansfield, Marx, and Rosenthal, 1989, p. M77). In their study of 408 LTC residents aged 70 to 99, Cohen-Mansfield, Marx, and Rosenthal, identified four principal types of agitation: aggressive, physically nonaggressive, verbal, and hiding/hoarding. The specific behaviors associated with each of these categories are listed in Table 7.1.

TABLE 7.1. Types of Agitation Identified in LTC Residents

- *Aggressive Behavior:* hitting, kicking, pushing, scratching, tearing things, cursing.
- *Physically Nonaggressive Behavior:* pacing, inappropriate robing or dis-robing, trying to get to a different place, restlessness, handling things inappropriately, repetitious mannerisms.
- *Verbally Agitated Behavior:* complaining, constant requests for attention, repetitious sentences/questions, negativism.
- *Hiding/Hoarding*

These authors found that agitation was a pervasive problem in LTC, as 93 percent of the residents showed one or more agitated behaviors at least once per week during the study. The authors concluded: "Despite the fact that the majority of these behaviors were nonaggressive and verbal, their sheer number is disconcerting, especially when one considers the effects that these behaviors have on other nursing home residents and personnel" (Cohen-Mansfield, Marx, and Rosenthal, 1989, p. M82).

In this section, we discuss interventions for four of the most common types of agitation: physical aggression and resistance to care, noisemaking, verbal abuse, and wandering.

Physical Aggression

Physical aggression is the most troublesome agitated behavior because of its potential for causing harm to the resident and others.

A recent study indicated that it is the most common reason for admission to a geropsychiatric hospital (Viewig et al., 1995). Intervening successfully with aggressive behavior in the LTC setting can not only help the resident to stay in the least restrictive environment, but also can save Medicare a great deal of money by avoiding hospitalization of aggressive residents.

Some causes of physical aggression are listed Table 7.2. These include external and internal triggers. External triggers can be care-related, control-related, or resident-related. Two of the internal triggers are ones that we discussed in the last section: misperceptions of others and hallucinations/delusions, which often go hand in hand.

Often, two or more of these triggers occur at the same time, leading to an aggressive outburst. For example, residents often misperceive (internal trigger) when caregiving (external trigger) is occurring.

TABLE 7.2. Possible Triggers for Physical Aggression

Internal Triggers

- Misperceptions of others
- Frustration caused by memory impairment or stroke-related hemiplegia/aphasia
- Hallucinations/delusions
- Physical problems and pain
- Fatigue

Care-Related Triggers

- Touching
- Shame at being showered or having a diaper changed
- The particular staff person doing the care

Control-Related Triggers

- Asking the person to change clothes or go to bed when she/he does not want to do so
- Stopping a person from going into a prohibited area
- Demanding too much of a patient

Resident-Related Triggers

- Wheelchair collisions
- Touching/pawing by a demented resident
- Another resident's yelling

Some possible interventions for various causes of aggression are listed in Table 7.3.

Finally, we should state the obvious: irritable staff often irritate irritable residents. Robinson, Spencer, and White (1989) underscore the importance of staff's demeanor in preventing angry outbursts:

A gentle, supportive, simple approach will almost always be more successful than commands or rationalizing. Dementia victims will often sense a caregiver's frustration or anger and become anxious or angry themselves. (p. A-3)

TABLE 7.3. Preventing and Minimizing Physical Aggression

Cause	Intervention
Care-related, control-related, or triggered by another	• Change antecedents • Prevent the other resident's behavior
Delusions, hallucinations, or misperceptions	• Minimize stimulation by moving slowly; approach resident from the front; reduce noise; and make minimal changes in routine (Hussian and Davis, 1985) • Psychiatric medication
Medical problem	• Treat problem
Attention	• Withdraw from client immediately when aggression starts, provide attention when resident is calm

Resistance to Care

Many residents resist staff during care through hitting and kicking, through pushing staff's arms away, or refusing to comply. Taylor, Ray, and Meador (1994) note several reasons that demented residents resist care: they (1) may feel "rushed or treated roughly," (2) may have "a fear of being dropped or treated poorly," (3) may be attempting to assert "control and reduce feelings of powerlessness," or (4) may believe staff are abusing them (p. 44).

To enhance cooperation during caregiving, these authors recommend several interventions (Taylor, Ray, and Meador, 1994). First, wherever possible, have the staff member with the best relationship with the patient provide care. Second, during the part of care that often triggers resistance, have another staff member keep the resident distracted. Third, allow the resident as much control as possible by providing her with choices and allowing her to use as many of her own skills as possible. Fourth, explain what you are doing, and if resistance occurs, explain it again. Finally, if the resident is using his hands to resist care, "put something in the person's hands, such as a washcloth or an interesting object" (Taylor, Ray, and Meador, 1994, p. 45). If resistance persists despite these interventions, they recommend that staff stop caregiving and try again later.

Birkett (1991) recommends that for resistive patients, staff should begin care with two aides present. In this way "one of them can serve as bodyguard and protect the other from blows or punches" (Birkett, 1991, p. 111). Once caregiving is under way, the second aide can leave because residents are less likely to be combative later on in the session.

When frustration is a trigger for a resident's aggression, we note Hussian and Davis' (1985) recommendation of light restraint. These authors describe this intervention as follows:

> Lightly restrain the client's arm or leg or other body part being used to strike out and gently ask the client to stop. Gradually reduce your contact until the episode subsides. (pp. 175-176)

Case Illustration

Mrs. B, an 82-year-old Caucasian female, had a diagnosis of Status-Post (S/P) Cerebral Vascular Accident (CVA), and exhibited minor cognitive impairment. She was incontinent of bladder and bowel and needed assistance with all ADLs. She resisted care from staff by hitting, grabbing staff, and yelling. Because of these problems, she was taking a low dose of Haldol.

As staff did a baseline assessment of her resistance to care, they noticed that prior to her aggressive outbursts, she became tense and fidgeted a great deal. As a result, they identified increasing tension as a trigger for her aggression. Staff then developed strategies for heading off this tension before it gained momentum. Specifically, they spoke in a soft voice when approaching her, used reassuring touch (with her permission), and always spent a few minutes prior to care sitting and talking with her until she appeared relaxed. Once care was underway and her temper flared, staff backed off and gave her a few minutes to calm down. A CNA who had the best rapport with Mrs. B was assigned to her regular care. This CNA allowed Mrs. B to do as much of her own care as possible, thus giving her an increased sense of control.

During a family conference, staff discovered that she loved to garden. They decided to use a wheelchair tour of the home's garden as a reinforcer for her compliance with care. Over the next few months, she gradually improved to the point where other staff could care for her without her having outbursts. Inspired by this success, the activities director arranged for volunteers to build elevated garden beds so that Mrs. B could spend sunny afternoons working with plants on the patio. Given these improvements, nursing staff could then talk with her physician about the possibility of reducing or discontinuing her Haldol.

Noisemaking

Noisemaking is one of the most psychologically taxing problems for staff and residents in LTC. Constant noisemaking can be very irritating to both staff and residents, and can trigger angry outbursts in other residents.

Ryan et al. (1988) found that about 30 percent of residents in LTC were noisemakers. Almost a third of the noisemaking was described as "purposeless and perseverative," because it had no specific trigger and was not reduced when staff provided attention. This type of noisemaking is often seen in residents with moderate to severe dementia who are seeking stimulation (Hussian, 1986). Ryan et al. (1988) also found that 27 percent of the noisemaking was caused by an internal or external trigger, such as caregiving, other residents, pain, or incontinence. About 18 percent of the noisemaking was designed to gain attention from staff. This type of noisemaking included "persistent calling for attention, complaining, or frequent loud demands" (Ryan et al., 1988, p. 370).

We have found that intervening with noisemakers is often very difficult when the primary cause is stimulation seeking. Here, staff should attempt obvious interventions, such as assuring that the person is wearing a hearing aid and that he is engaged in as many activities as possible. Staff can also ask the family to bring the resident a tape player and tapes of his favorite music.

In cases where noisemaking is caused by internal or external triggers, staff can design interventions to prevent the triggers. For example, if a resident's need for toileting is a trigger for yelling, staff can schedule the resident for toileting at regular intervals of perhaps two hours. This prevents the activator (need for toileting) from occurring spontaneously, provides the resident with attention when she is not agitated, and provides her with consistent contact with staff, which may reassure her of their availability (Fatis, Smasal, and Betts, 1989).

In cases where attention seeking is the cause, staff should use the "ignore and attend" strategy that we have discussed before: ignoring the repetitive complaints and demands for attention and giving attention when the resident is quiet. A problem with this approach is that staff often provide attention reflexively to a resident's cry of distress or complaint, which reinforces the noisemaking. Even if a minority of staff respond to inappropriate complaints and demands, the behavior is "intermittently reinforced," making it more resistant to elimination. For this reason, before starting this intervention, all staff should be thoroughly trained in the procedure and should be told the specific type of noisemaking to ignore.

Case Illustration

Mrs. P, a 72-year-old Caucasian female, was admitted with diagnoses of Chronic Obstructive Pulmonary Disease (COPD) and alcohol and valium abuse. A former office clerk, she had divorced 12 years prior and had no children or other relatives to visit her. Mrs. P had poor vision even when wearing her glasses, and displayed minor cognitive impairment, including a deficit in recent memory.

Mrs. P refused to use her call light, and instead, yelled for the nurses throughout the day. When the nurses came, she could not tell them what she wanted. Consequently, staff began to ignore Mrs. P, which, in turn, escalated her calling out.

She was evaluated by the mental health consultant, who recommended a hearing evaluation. Once Mrs. P was fitted with hearing aids, the volume of her yelling decreased immediately. The consultant also recommended that staff use behavioral interventions that would address her need for attention and reassurance.

The staff tried a number of behavioral interventions. They provided Mrs. P with lots of attention when she was quiet and used her call light. They moved her to a room directly across from the nurses' station, where she could see staff and receive frequent, reassuring comments. The nurses brought her in her wheelchair to the nurses' station whenever possible. The activities director interviewed her about her lifelong interests, which included country-western music. The director then arranged for a donation of a tape player and music tapes from a local charity. After six weeks of using these interventions, the frequency of her yelling decreased, and she expressed increased satisfaction with her treatment at the home.

Verbal Abuse

Verbal abuse is often directed at staff during caregiving because residents with dementia often misinterpret what staff are doing. Another cause of verbal abuse is the irritability that often accompanies depression.

Intervening with verbally abusive residents requires the same analysis as for other problem behaviors: identifying triggers and reinforcing consequences. Is the verbal abuse triggered by physical discomfort, delusions and hallucinations, or depression and irritability? Is one particular person, type of person (e.g., male or female), or type of care more likely to trigger verbal abuse? Are staff withdrawing from a verbally abusive resident, making it more likely that she will increase her verbal abuse to get more attention? Answers to questions like these will guide your interventions.

Lichtenberg (1994) describes a case in which the "ignore and attend" intervention was used with a 69-year-old verbally abusive, cognitively intact woman. This woman, Mrs. O, constantly belittled the staff and made inappropriate requests. The following intervention was used:

A behavioral contract was written outlining what responsibilities the staff had and what Mrs. O's responsibilities were. When Mrs. O became verbally hostile, the staff was instructed to respond, "Mrs. O, I cannot work with you when you are verbally hostile. I will return in ten minutes to try to work with you again." As a result of the plan, Mrs. O's hostilities diminished greatly, and she began to meet more of her own needs. (p. 96)

Wandering

Wandering is a problem when residents venture into others' rooms, into off-limits areas, or outside the facility. Some wanderers are goal-directed (e.g., going home, finding the bathroom), whereas others have no destination and are wandering to gain stimulation (Algase, 1993). Hussian and Davis (1985) point out that wanderers who seek stimulation through wandering often exhibit other kinds of self-stimulation such as door knob rattling, clapping, rocking, rubbing themselves, or patting things. In the case of one of our residents, a wanderer grabbed patients' wheelchair handles tightly and would not let go.

For wanderers seeking stimulation, at least two interventions can be tried. First, provide exercise so the resident can gain stimulation from an activity other than wandering. Staff may have to provide individual exercise sessions for residents who cannot focus on group exercise activities. Second, Hussian and Davis (1985) suggest providing a variety of inedible items that can be squeezed, rubbed, or shaken. For example, a teddy bear, PlayDoh™, or Silly Putty™ could be used.

For wanderers who are looking for the bathroom because they forget where it is, staff can place a picture of a toilet on the door, label the door, or paint it a bright color (Robinson et al., 1989). Similarly, for wanderers who cannot recall where their room is, their room door can be marked with a bright color, a picture of themselves, or a name plate. Hermann (1992) provides the following example of how such a method was used to train a resident who could not find her room:

A large brightly coloured disk was placed on Mrs. E's door, and she was trained to direct her attention to it. Each time a staff member accompanied her to her room they pointed out the disk. When she was found in other residents' rooms, the staff showed her that there was no disk on the door. After several weeks, this simple behavioral intervention reduced her tendency to wander into other rooms. (p. 55)

For wanderers who are trying to exit the building, to enter off-limits areas, or to enter other residents' rooms, a brightly colored visual barrier is often helpful. This visual barrier is about 24" high and spans the width of the doorway. It can be fastened with Velcro™, which makes it easy to remove and replace when people enter and exit the area. The effectiveness of such a barrier was recently tested in a dementia care unit by Dickinson, McLain-Kark, and Marshall-Baker (1995). They found that it reduced residents' attempts to exit a dementia care unit by 96 percent. Visual barriers like this one are available through nursing home supply catalogs.

Case Illustation

Mr. M, a 78-year-old Hispanic male with Alzheimer's dementia, was admitted because he had increasingly wandered away from his board and care home. While he was bilingual, Spanish was his first language, and he often reverted back to speaking only Spanish. He was a devout Catholic who was quite active in his church. His medical diagnoses were arthritis and prostrate cancer, in remission. He was oriented only to person.

While at the nursing home, he continued to wander, and thus staff were considering a transfer to an Alzheimer's unit. Mr. M wandered out of the building as well as into others' rooms, where he indiscriminately picked up knickknacks and other small objects. Baseline assessment showed that he was most likely to wander in the late afternoon and when he needed toileting. Both staff and his family members were reluctant to use restraints, though they did use a geri-chair in the late afternoons. Because need for toileting was also a trigger for wandering, Mr. M was placed on a two-hour toileting program.

Staff also intervened in a number of other creative ways. They assigned Spanish-speaking staff to care for him. They noted which rooms he frequented most often and, using Velcro™, installed 24" yellow bands across the doorways. To help him identify his room, they installed a large green circle (his favorite color) on his door and over his bed. They also noticed that the back door was his favorite escape route, so they installed a red stop sign on it, which proved effective. To deter him from taking small objects, the activities director had his family bring in a box of stuffed animals, trinkets, and blocks for him to use as he wished. To promote exercise and to help him use up energy, staff arranged for him to go on walks supervised by volunteers from his church. When he left the building unattended, staff were instructed to walk with him until he could be easily directed back in. These interventions proved so effective that the geri-chair was no longer needed and transfer to an Alzheimer's unit was avoided.

SEXUAL PROBLEMS

We see two types of inappropriate sexual behavior in LTC: masturbation in public areas, and fondling or sexual contact at inappropriate times and places. Sexual contact between residents may or may not be appropriate, depending upon whether they have both consented or are capable of consenting.

Before we address these issues, we must be clear about our own values. First, old age and sex are not incompatible, and sex may be a great source of enjoyment well into old age. Second, sexual contact between two residents must be consensual. Staff should err on the side of preventing exploitation rather than on the side of sexual permissiveness. However, once mutual consent has been obtained, staff should take a proactive role in providing residents with privacy for sexual expression. Third, confidentiality about the residents' consensual sexual behavior should be maintained wherever possible.

We believe that staff members' values about sexual expression affect how they deal with sexual issues in LTC. At one extreme are staff who are embarrassed by sexual expression. These staff members may respond by ignoring a problem and hoping that it will go away, or by strictly prohibiting all sexual contact. At the other extreme are staff who appreciate the sexual needs of residents, but who permit it even in situations where mutual consent has not been established. We hope that you will find the middle ground between these positions. We could call this middle ground the "enlightened but cautious approach" to sexuality in LTC.

Assessing Competency for Consensual Sexual Contact

How can we tell whether a resident is capable of consenting to sexual contact so that exploitation by another resident is avoided? Lichtenberg (1994) has created the guidelines listed in Table 7.4. As you can see, the first step is to administer the Mini-Mental State Exam. If the resident scores 14 or below, she is deemed incapable of consenting and sexual contact is not permitted. If she scores 15 or above, an interview is conducted to explore the resident's awareness of the relationship, her ability to avoid exploitation, and her awareness of potential risks. The key questions assessed during this interview are also listed in Table 7.4.

Once the interview is completed, the results are analyzed. Regarding protection from exploitation, the resident is judged incompetent if she "appears unable to set the limits" with her partner, or thinks that she "must always submit to sexual demands" (Lichtenberg, 1994, p. 147). Regarding awareness of the relationship, if the resident thinks that her partner is a long-term spouse or denies the relationship, she would be seen as incompetent. While awareness of risks in the relationship is desirable, Dr. Lichtenberg does not believe it is essential for competence. However, he does emphasize that staff should frequently remind the resident of the risks.

Once this analysis is concluded, the results are presented to the interdisciplinary team. At this meeting, staff "provide feedback on any behavioral evidence that supported or contradicted the patient's responses" (Lichtenberg, 1994, p. 148). A final decision is then made about the patient's competency for intimacy.

If a resident with dementia is found competent, Dr. Lichtenberg recommends informing the family about this decision, though he admits that this is difficult. Specifically, the family should be told of the resident's sexual interest and about the evaluation process that staff have used to establish her competence. If the family has objections, they are invited to discuss them with the treatment team. However, "unless the family can share behavioral observations that contradict the assessment findings, the team will allow the romantic relationship to continue" (Lichtenberg, 1994, p. 148).

TABLE 7.4. Decision Tree for Assessing Competency to Participate in a Sexual Relationship

Areas to Assess and Questions	Action
1. *Cognitive impairment:* Does the resident score 15 or more on the Mini-Mental State Exam?	If yes: interview resident. If no: resident incompetent.
2. *Potential for exploitation:* Does resident know who the other person is and which of them is initiating sexual contact? Can the resident state what level of intimacy he is comfortable with?	If yes: continue interview. If no: resident is incompetent.
3. *Awareness of the relationship:* Is the behavior consistent with resident's formerly held values? Can the resident reject uninvited sexual contact?	If yes: continue interview. If no: resident is incompetent.
4. *Awareness of risk:* Does the resident realize the relationship may be time-limited? Can the resident describe how she will react when the relationship ends?	If yes: resident is competent. If no: provide frequent reminders of risks, but permit relationship.

Source: Adapted from Lichtenberg (1994). Used by permission of Haworth Press, Inc. and Dr. Lichtenberg.

Of course, for cognitively intact residents whose physician has deemed them capable of making their own medical decisions, their right to confidentiality must be respected. Our opinion is that staff should not discuss the sexual practices of these residents with the family unless they give permission.

Intervening with Sexually Inappropriate Behavior

There are two types of inappropriate sexual behavior: masturbating in public and sexually touching staff or nonconsenting residents. With both types of behavior, staff should usually do a behavioral tracking over time to rule out external and internal triggers for the behavior. Staff can then design interventions that prevent the trigger, or they can try one of the interventions described below.

Residents who masturbate in public areas usually do not realize that this is an inappropriate place to do so. As a result, the strategy used by Hussian and Davis (1985) is to teach a resident that the appropriate place for masturbation is in his room. To do so, they place a large, bright-colored disc or cloth above his bed. When he masturbates in a public area, staff "take the resident before the activity is completed into his room, point to the color cue and allow the behavior to continue" (Hussian and Davis, 1985, p. 180). Since taking him to his room may not be possible on every occasion, staff can interrupt the masturbation or use light restraint in lieu of taking him to his room. By discouraging it every time it "occurs in the wrong setting and allowing it to continue in the right setting, the exposure or masturbation should begin to occur only in the designated areas" (Hussian and Davis, 1985, p. 180).

When the behavior involves fondling staff, there are a number of options. If the resident does it during care with opposite-sex staff members, same-sex staff members could be substituted, or vice versa. Alternatively, staff can leave the room immediately and resume care later on. Sometimes using two aides rather than one is helpful. Obviously, staff should provide praise when the resident cooperates and is nonabusive.

When the unwanted or inappropriate sexual touching is directed toward a resident, staff should focus their efforts on decreasing opportunities for contact between the two. If the resident is entering another's room and fondling her, staff can place a visual barrier, such as the orange cloth described earlier in this chapter, over the door of the target resident's room. If the target is a roommate, staff may need to move one of the residents or place the perpetrator in a private room.

Medication

If these behavioral interventions do not work, the attending physician or your psychotropic medication committee can consider medication as a last resort. Tranquilizers and antilibidinal drugs are two that physicians often prescribe.

One antilibidinal drug is Depo Provera (Medroxyprogesterone Acetate), which decreases a man's sex drive by lowering his body's production of testosterone (Cooper, 1987). Psychiatrist A.J. Cooper, MD, gave Depo Provera to four elderly men with mild to moderate dementia who demonstrated inappropriate sexual behavior. The men's sexual behavior included "compulsive masturbation, genital exposure, and attempts to fondle and engage in coitus with female residents" (Cooper, 1987, p. 369). During the 12 months that they received this medication, the sexual behavior was eliminated. After they were taken off the medication, three of the four men continued to refrain from inappropriate behavior over the next 12 months.

The potential side effects of Depo Provera include symptoms such as weight gain, lethargy, hyperglycemia, hypogonadism, nightmares, leg cramps, insomnia, headache, and hot and cold flashes (Gottesman and Schubert, 1993). Cooper (1987) cautions that some of these side effects are very difficult to detect in demented residents. To detect and prevent these, he emphasizes that it is necessary to use "scrupulous physician and staff observations, supplemented by laboratory testing" (p. 370). However, he argues that, when compared with tranquilizers, Depo Provera is safer and has fewer potential adverse side effects.

The problem with Dr. Cooper's study is that it did not use a control group. We have not found a controlled study that has used a population of demented elderly men who demonstrate sexually inappropriate behavior. A few studies have evaluated Depo Provera's effectiveness with sex offenders (Kravitz et al., 1995) and mentally retarded sex offenders (Cooper, 1995). However, until more studies are done with our population, we should withhold firm judgement about its efficacy for elderly men.

An additional concern is that the use of antilibidinal agents raises serious ethical issues, because they impinge directly on personal freedom. Consequently, Cooper (1987) emphasizes that informed consent from the resident or the signing family member must be obtained. We add that staff should consider having their Bioethics Committee (see Chapter 10) discuss this issue and make recommendations on a case-by-case basis.

Case Study

Mr. Z, an 81-year-old male of German descent, was admitted with his wife, with whom he shared a room. His diagnoses included S/P CVA, diabetes, and hypertension. He was incontinent of bowel, exhibited mild cognitive impairment, and needed assistance with most ADLs. He was not taking psychiatric medication.

Mr. Z was referred to the social services consultant because of inappropriate masturbation, which occurred in the lobby and always within view of his wife. When she saw him masturbating there, she became angry and belittled him. Further assessment revealed that the couple had long-standing marital conflicts and that the wife had been the dominant spouse. In response to his wife's attempts to control him, Mr. Z typically responded in a passive/aggressive way.

To begin with, Mr. and Mrs. Z were moved to separate rooms on a trial basis. Marital counseling was recommended through the mental health consultant. The social services consultant drew up a written agreement with Mr. Z that he would not masturbate in public areas. To remind him of this agreement, the consultant placed a blue ribbon on the arm of his wheelchair. The staff often reminded him of the agreement and constantly praised his compliance. While the long-standing marital conflicts were not resolved, the behavior ceased and the separate rooms proved beneficial to both residents.

DEPRESSION TREATED WITH BEHAVIOR THERAPY

We briefly referred to Behavior Therapy in Chapter 5 when we discussed theories of psychotherapy. Therapists who treat depression with Behavior Therapy believe that mood is directly influenced by our participation in pleasant activities. Studies (e.g., Lewinsohn and Graff, 1973) have shown that the fewer the pleasant activities that someone participates in, the more likely he is to be depressed.

According to this school of thought, we can best intervene with a depressed resident by helping him to increase his participation in pleasant activities.

What makes this challenging is that depressed people often say they "don't feel like doing anything." In these cases, we hope to get them to do at least a very small activity each day that will break up their lethargy and get the ball rolling, however slowly.

Teri and Logsdon (1991) describe pleasant activities for patients with dementia, and some of these are listed in Table 7.5. Because some of these mood-elevating activities occur routinely in LTC, it is easy for us to overlook the fact that they can have a decidedly positive effect on mood. Even minor activities such as self-grooming and recalling past events can help to enhance a resident's mood on a given day. Of course, these activities should be tailored to the resident's interests.

TABLE 7.5. Pleasant Activities for LTC Residents

- *Interactive:* Visiting with or having meals with family and friends, being with pets, getting/sending letters and cards, going on outings, being complimented or told I am loved, playing games, recalling and discussing past events.

- *Recreational:* Listening to stories or poems, listening to music, watching TV or movies, doing puzzles or crosswords, eating snacks, attending church services, reading or watching news, doing handwork, exercising, indoor gardening, looking at photo albums, singing.

- *Others:* Grooming self, being outside, napping, wearing certain clothes.

When it comes to addressing specific symptoms of depression in demented residents, Teri and Gallagher-Thompson (1991) describe several behavioral interventions, some of which are listed in Table 7.6. In our experience, one that is particularly effective is to have family members visit at mealtime if the resident is eating poorly. In several cases, the resident has begun eating more once the family started visiting during meals.

INSOMNIA

Insomnia may be caused by physical or mental problems, or both. One common medical cause is sleep-disordered breathing (e.g., sleep apnea), which can be treated with various interventions such as weight loss, avoidance of sedatives, and surgery (Neylan, De May, and Reynolds, 1996). Another is periodic leg movements or restless leg syndrome, which can be treated with medication (Neylan, De May, and Reynolds, 1996).

TABLE 7.6. Interventions for Depressed Residents with Alzheimer's Disease

Problem	*Possible Interventions*
Eating poorly	• Praise resident for eating. • Pair eating with concurrent pleasant activity, such as visits from relatives.
Insomnia	• Increase regular exercise and activities. • Decrease stimulants.
Feelings of worthlessness	• Encourage pleasant reminiscing about the past.
Loss of interest	• Increase pleasant activities. • Gear activities to cognitive level.

Source: Teri and Gallagher-Thompson, 1991.

Concerning mental disorders associated with insomnia, anxiety and depression are the most prominent. Two behavioral interventions for insomnia are mentioned in Table 7.6. Another intervention is playing a relaxation tape for the resident at bedtime.

In intervening with insomnia, a common question is whether daytime napping causes nighttime insomnia. If a resident has trouble sleeping at night, should she be encouraged not to nap during the day? A study by Regestein and Morris (1987) suggests that the answer may be "no" for some residents. These authors investigated whether daytime napping really is associated with nocturnal insomnia. Their study involved 16 female LTC residents aged 73 to 100 who did not have a sleep problem, were not taking psychiatric medications, and displayed mild-moderate cognitive impairment. The results were surprising: the more these residents slept during the day, the more they slept at night, and the less they slept during the day, the less they slept at night. Thus, daytime napping did not interfere with nighttime sleep. The implication is that for residents who suffer from insomnia, denying a daytime nap may not enhance their nighttime sleep.

Of course, each resident's particular circumstances have to be evaluated before a conclusion can be reached. It is often helpful to have the staff track the length and frequency of napping and the length of time that she sleeps at night. This may show whether there is a relationship between the two.

CONCLUSION

In this chapter we have attempted to park as many practical suggestions as we can under one roof. In applying these in our own LTC facilities, we have had to use a trial-and-error, hypothesis-testing approach. Sometimes one works and another does not; sometimes nothing works. Regardless, the more interventions that we can choose from and apply, the greater our chance of success.

Because applying these interventions effectively can be complicated, staff should ask advice from their mental health consultant wherever possible. Even if the insurance company or physician has refused to authorize an evaluation, staff can still discuss a case briefly with the consultant and ask for specific interventions. As they use the trial-and-error method, staff can ask for further advice as the case unfolds.

Of course, even fine-tuned behavioral assessments and interventions do not always work. In such cases, staff must often consider the option of psychotropic medications, which we discuss in the next chapter.

REFERENCES

Algase, D.L. (1993). Wandering: Assessment and intervention. In P. Szwabo and G. Grossberg (Eds.), *Problem behaviors in long-term care: Recognition, diagnosis, and treatment*. New York: Springer.

American Psychiatric Association (1994). *Diagnostic and statistical manual of mental disorders*, fourth edition. Washington: American Psychiatric Association.

Birkett, D.P. (1991). *Psychiatry in the nursing home: Assessment, evaluation, and intervention*. Binghamton, NY: The Haworth Press.

Carstenson, L.L. and Fremouw, W.J. (1981). The demonstration of a behavioral intervention for late life paranoia. *The Gerontologist, 21*, 329-333.

Christison, C., Christison, G., and Blazer, D.G. (1989). Late-life schizophrenia and paranoid disorders. In E.W. Busse and D.G. Blazer (Eds.), *Geriatric psychiatry* (pp. 403-414). Washington, DC: American Psychiatric Press.

Cohen-Mansfield, J., Marx, M.S., and Rosenthal, A.S. (1989). A description of agitation in a nursing home. *Journal of Gerontology,* 1989, *44* (3), 77-84.

Cooper, A.J. (1987). Medroxyprogesterone acetate (MPA) treatment of sexual acting out in men suffering from dementia. *Journal of Clinical Psychiatry, 48,* 368-370.

Cooper, A.J. (1995). Review of the role of two antilibidinal drugs in the treatment of sex offenders with mental retardation. *Mental Retardation, 33,* 42-48.

Curlik, S.M., Frazier, D., and Katz, I.R. (1991). Psychiatric aspects of long-term care. In J. Sadavoy, L. Lazarus, and L. Jarvik (Eds.), *Comprehensive review of geriatric psychiatry* (pp. 547-564). Washington, DC: American Psychiatric Press.

Dickinson, J.I., McLain-Kark, J., and Marshall-Baker, A. (1995). The effects of visual barriers on exiting behavior in a dementia care unit. *The Gerontologist, 35,* 127-130.

Fatis, M., Smasal, M.S., and Betts, B.J. (1989). Behavioral psychological intervention. *Journal of Gerontological Nursing, 15* (1), 25-28.

Gottesman, H.G. and Schubert, D.S.P. (1993). Low-dose oral Medroxyprogesterone Acetate in the management of the paraphilias. *Journal of Clinical Psychiatry, 54,* 182-188.

Hermann, N. (1992). Dementia. In D. Conn, N. Herrmann, A. Kaye, D. Rewilak, A. Robinson, and B. Schogt (Eds.), *Practical psychiatry in the nursing home: A handbook for staff* (pp. 43-62). Seattle: Hoegrefe and Huber.

Hussian, R.A. (1986). Severe behavioral problems. In L. Teri and P. Lewinsohn (Eds.), *Geropsychological assessment and treatment.* New York: Springer.

Hussian, R.A. and Davis, R.L. (1985). *Responsive care: Behavioral interventions with elderly persons.* Champaign, IL: Research Press.

Koening, H.G., Christison, C., Christison, G., and Blazer, D.G. (1996). Schizophrenia and paranoid disorders. In E.W. Busse and D.G. Blazer (Eds.), *The American Psychiatric Press textbook of geriatric psychiarty,* (pp. 265-278). Washington, DC: American Psychiatric Press.

Kravitz, H.M., Haywood, T.W., Kelly, J., Wahlstrom, C., Liles, S., and Cavanaugh, J.L. (1995). Medroxyprogesterone treatment for paraphiliacs. *Bulletin of the American Academy of Psychiatry and Law, 23,* 19-33.

Lewinsohn, P.M. and Graff, M. (1973). Pleasant activities and depression. *Journal of Consulting and Clinical Psychology, 41,* 261-268.

Lichtenberg, P.A. (1994). *A guide to psychological practice in geriatric long-term care.* Binghamton, NY: The Haworth Press.

Neylan, T.C., De May, M.G., and Reynolds, C.F. (1996). Sleep and chronobiological disturbances. In E.W. Busse and D.G. Blazer (Eds.), *The American Psychiatric Press textbook of geriatric psychiatry,* 2nd Edition (pp. 329-340). Washington, DC: American Psychiatric Press.

Regestein, Q.R. and Morris, J. (1987). Daily sleep patterns observed among institutionalized elderly residents. *Journal of the American Geriatric Society, 35,* 767-772.

Robinson, A., Spencer, B., and White, L. (1989). *Understanding difficult behaviors: Some practical suggestions for coping with Alzheimer's Disease and related illnesses.* Eastern Michigan University, Ann Arbor, Michigan: Geriatric Education Center of Michigan.

Ryan, D.P., Tainsh, S.M.M., Kolodny, V., Lendrum, B.L., and Fisher, R.H. (1988). Noise-making amongst the elderly in long-term care. *The Gerontologist, 28,* 369-371.

Shuchter, S.R. and Zisook, S. (1993). The course of normal grief. In M.S. Stroebe, W. Stroebe, and R.O. Hansson (Eds.), *Handbook of bereavement: Theory, research, and intervention.* New York: Cambridge University Press.

Taylor, J.A., Ray, W.A., and Meador, K.G. (1994). *Managing behavioral symptoms in nursing home residents: A manual for nursing home staff.* Nashville: Vanderbilt University School of Medicine. (Available from the Health Standards and Quality Bureau, Health Care Financing Administration, 7500 Security Bl., Baltimore MD 21244.)

Teri, L. and Logsdon, R.G. (1991). Identifying pleasant activities for Alzheimer's disease patients: The pleasant events schedule-AD. *The Gerontologist, 31*, 124-127.

Teri, L. and Gallagher-Thompson, D. (1991). Cognitive behavioral interventions for treatment of depression in Alzheimer's patients. *The Gerontologist, 31*, 413-416.

Viewig, V., Blair, C.E., Tucker, R., and Lewis, R. (1995). A geropsychiatric hospital survey to determine behavioral factors leading to hospital admission. *Journal of Clinical Geropsychology, 1*, 305-311.

Chapter 8

Psychiatric Medication

While ideally every LTC facility would have a geropsychiatrist or psychiatrist to prescribe and monitor psychiatric medications, few do. Consequently, the resident's attending physician usually prescribes all of the psychiatric medications as best he can. Unless this physician has had adequate training in psychopharmacology, the medications chosen may be less than optimal. The physician often depends upon the advice of nursing staff or the mental health consultant, who may or may not be well informed. While the prescribed medications and dosages are often monitored by a pharmacy consultant, this person also may not have in-depth training in psychopharmacology. As a result of these factors, the quality of psychiatric medicating in LTC facilities varies a great deal.

While only the attending physician can legally prescribe medication, in daily practice it is often the nursing staff who call her to ask for a certain medication. Under these circumstances, it is important that not only the nursing staff, but also the social services staff, be acquainted with the basics of psychiatric medication. Ideally, both disciplines would discuss basic medication options, rather than having the decision made solely by nursing. This is especially true when it is the social services designee who has most carefully assessed the resident's mental and behavioral functioning.

The purpose of this chapter is to provide a brief and basic overview of the major types of psychiatric medications and their common side effects. We also discuss screening for tardive dyskinesia, a potentially irreversible problem for residents taking antipsychotic medications.

MAJOR TYPES OF PSYCHIATRIC MEDICATIONS AND THEIR SIDE EFFECTS

The five major types of psychiatric medications are: antipsychotics, antianxiety medications, sleep medications, antidepressants, and antimanic medications. Table 8.1 lists common medications from each of these categories. Note that some of the antimanic medications are also anticonvulsants used to prevent seizures.

There are five main side effects of psychiatric medications: sedation, orthostatic hypotension, anticholinergic effects, akathisia, and extrapyramidal effects. *Sedation* can be caused by all five types of medication, though some medications are much more sedating than others. The greater the sedation, the more likely a resident is to experience temporary cognitive impairment, such as poor concentration and memory of recent events. *Orthostatic hypotension*, a drop in blood pressure related to postural changes such as rising from a chair or bed, may be caused by certain antipsychotic, antianxiety, anti-depressant, or sleep medications. This side effect is of particular concern in the elderly because it places them at greater risk of falling (Hermann, 1992). Antidepressant medications which minimize sedation and orthostatic hypotension include Prozac, Paxil, Zoloft, and Wellbutrin (Stoudemire, Moran, and Fogel, 1995). An antianxiety medication that minimizes sedation is Buspar, a nonbenzodiazepine (Cole and Yonkers, 1995). Ambien (Zolpidem), also a nonbenzodiazepine, is a sleep medication that does not cause daytime sedation or memory problems (Neylan, De May, and Reynolds, 1996).

Anticholinergic side effects are associated with some antipsychotic and antidepressant medications, and include the following problems: dry mouth, blurred vision, constipation, urinary retention, tachycardia, and delirium (Wise and Rundell, 1995). Anticholinergic medications are of particular concern in the elderly because they may impair memory and may trigger delirium. Consequently, it is important for LTC staff to know which antidepressants and antipsychotics are least anticholinergic. Some of these are listed in Table 8.2.

Akathisia, associated with antipsychotic medications, involves "motor restlessness in which the resident feels compelled to keep moving or pacing" (Hermann, 1992, p. 188). At times, a patient with akathisia may not display movement outwardly, but inwardly may feel extremely uncomfortable because of feelings of restlessness.

Finally, *extrapyramidal symptoms*, such as dystonias and parkinsonism, may be caused by antipsychotic medications (Bezchlibnyk-Butler, Jeffries, and Martin, 1994). *Dystonias*, which rarely occur

TABLE 8.1. Common Psychiatric Medications

Antipsychotic Medications

Clozaril (clozapine)
Mellaril (thioridazine)
Navane (thiothixene)
Risperdal (risperidone)
Thorazine (chlorpromazine)

Haldol (haloperidol)
Loxitane (loxapine)
Prolixin (fluphenazine)
Stelazine (trifluoperazine)
Trilafon (perphenazine)

Antianxiety and Sedative Medications

Benzodiazepines

Ativan (lorazepam)
Librium (chlordiazepoxide)
Klonopin (clonazepam)
Serax (oxazepam)
Valium (diazepam)
Xanax(alprazolam)

Nonbenzodiazepines

Atarax, Vistaril (hydroxyzine)
Benadryl (dephenhydramine)
Chloral Hydrate
Buspar (buspirone)

Medications for Sleep

Benzodiazepines

Restoril (temazepam)
Halcion (triazolam)
Desyrel (trazodone)

Nonbenzodiazepines

Ambien (zolpidem)
Benadryl (diphenhydramine)

Antidepressants

Asendin (amoxapine)
Desyrel (trazodone)
Norpramine (desipramine)
Paxil (paroxetine)
Sinequan (doxepin)
Wellbutrin (buproprion)

Anafranil (clomipramine)
Aventyl (nortriptyline)
Elavil (amitriptyline)
Pamelor (nortriptyline)
Prozac (fluoxetine)
Tofranil (imipramine)
Zoloft (sertraline)

Antimanic and Anticonvulsant Medications

Lithium Carbonate
Depakene (valproate)

Tegretol (carbamazepine)
Gabapentin

TABLE 8.2. Some Antipsychotic and Antidepressant Medications Associated with Fewer Anticholinergic Side Effects

Antipsychotic Medications

Haldol (haloperidol)	Risperdal (risperidone)
Stelazine (trifluoperazine)	

Antidepressants

Desyrel (trazodone)	Norpramine (desipramine)
Prozac (fluoxetine)	Wellbutrin (bupropion)
Zoloft (sertraline)	

Source: Stoudemire, Moran, and Fogel, 1995; Bezchlibnyk-Butler, Jeffries, and Martin, 1994.

in the elderly, consist of "acute, sustained contractions" of the muscles of the mouth, neck, and eyes (Hermann, 1992, p. 187). These are often treated with immediate intramuscular injections of a medication such as Benadryl or Cogentin. *Parkinsonism* involves symptoms similar to those of Parkinson's disease, including muscular stiffness and rigidity, tremor, an expressionless face, and/or shuffling when walking (Bezchlibnyk-Butler, Jeffries, and Martin, 1994). Elderly female residents are particularly vulnerable to the effects of parkinsonism and akathisia (Bezchlibnyk-Butler, Jeffries, and Martin, 1994). Parkinsonism is usually treated with antiparkinsonian agents, such as Artane or Cogentin, which relieve much of the rigidity and tremor (Bezchlibnyk-Butler, Jeffries, and Martin, 1994). However, these medications are also quite anticholinergic, and residents taking them must be monitored for this type of side effect. Note that residents taking both an antipsychotic medication *and* a medication for its side effects receive anticholinergic side effects from two sources.

HCFA (1995) guidelines require that residents taking antipsychotic medication be monitored for the above side effects. If a resident displays pronounced side effects, the attending physician may change medications, lower the dose, or prescribe an additional medication to help control these.

Risperdal (risperidone)

We pause here to highlight a relatively new antipsychotic medication, Risperdal (risperidone). This medication is especially relevant to an LTC population because it has a lower rate of extra-pyramidal side effects than other antipsychotic medications like Haldol, especially "at low-to-moderate doses" (Mendelowitz and Lieberman, 1995, p. 4). Furthermore, when it comes to treating psychotic symptoms, risperidone is more effective than Haldol (Ereshefsky, 1995).

While risperidone has not been systematically tested with LTC patients, successful case studies and uncontrolled group studies have been reported. These group studies have shown decreased behavioral disturbances in demented, elderly patients treated with risperidone (Mendelowitz and Lieberman, 1995). There were also minimal extrapyramidal side effects in these patients. Fortunately, there is a national multisite study underway which is testing risperidone with this population.

Tardive Dyskinesia

Another way in which antipsychotic medication can affect muscular movement is through tardive dyskinesia (TD). TD involves potentially irreversible, involuntary movements caused by taking antipsychotic medication. The primary symptoms are oral and facial, including any of the following: protrusion or twisting of the tongue, lip smacking, pursing and sucking of the lips, chewing and lateral jaw motions, and cheek puffing (APA Task Force, 1992). Other symptoms can involve abnormal, involuntary movements of the neck, trunk, feet and hands (APA Task Force, 1992). TD usually occurs after three months or more on antipsychotic medication, but the elderly are particularly at risk for developing symptoms much earlier than that (APA Task Force, 1992).

These symptoms are different from "side effects," which occur only when the drug is given. TD may continue even after all medication is stopped and may never remit. This possibility of irreversible TD is one reason why antipsychotic medications are so risky. Another reason is that most LTC residents who take these medications have never taken them before, which places them at greater risk for TD. As Salzman, Satlin, and Burrows put it, "In elderly people who have not been previously treated with neuroleptics, tardive dyskinesia develops rapidly and at lower doses than with younger patients" (1995, p. 806).

Given these risks, psychiatrist Nathan Hermann, MD, makes the following recommendations for preventing TD in LTC residents:

1. avoid the use of neuroleptics if possible,
2. reduce and discontinue the [antipsychotic] medication as soon as possible following amelioration of symptomatology, and
3. examine each resident receiving a neuroleptic regularly to determine if there is any evidence of abnormal involuntary movements. (1992, p. 188)

To examine residents for TD, we recommend that you use standardized rating scales such as the Abnormal Involuntary Movement Scale (AIMS) or the Dyskinesia Identification System: Condensed User Scale (DISCUS). These instruments give you a score that indicates the possible presence or absence of TD. They can be given by nonmedical as well as medical staff members, provided they have been trained in using the scales. It is particularly easy to train staff to use the DISCUS because a videotaped training program is available (Kalachnik, Sprague, and Kalies, 1991). The manual that accompanies this program gives helpful suggestions about the assessment of TD and actions to take when a resident tests positive.

When a resident is about to be placed on an antipsychotic medication, it is a good idea to get a baseline score for TD prior to starting the medication (APA Task Force, 1992). Because abnormal movements may be present in residents who are not taking antipsychotic medication, this baseline score may prove helpful later on in deciding if a positive TD score is caused by the medication or was already present. Given that TD can begin within the first three months of taking antipsychotic medication, it is a good idea to do the next TD screening within those three months. Thereafter, residents "should be examined regularly, at least every three to six months, for early signs of TD" (APA Task Force, 1992, p. 249).

If you obtain a positive TD score for a resident, it is a good idea to do a reliability check by having another staff person assess that resident to see if his score is close to yours. Even if both scores are positive for signs of TD, that does not necessarily mean that TD is present because abnormal movements may have other medical causes other than antipsychotic medications (APA Task Force, 1992). As the APA Task Force puts it:

> Assessment techniques are important for identifying possible cases as well as documenting their severity and measuring treatment response or long-term outcome, but a process of clinical evaluation and differential diagnosis is necessary to establish the presence of TD. (1992, p. 235)

They emphasize that after a positive score, "a diagnostic evaluation should take place to rule out other neuromedical causes" (APA Task Force, 1992, p. 249). Kalachnik, Sprague, and Kalies (1991) note that the attending physician is responsible for doing this evaluation, and they describe an extensive protocol for her doing so.

If the physician decides that the resident does have Tardive Dyskinesia, he must decide what steps to take. The APA Task Force points out that "there remains no proven safe and effective treatment for TD" (1992, p. 237). However, stopping the medication often does help, as "33 to 50 percent of TD cases will dissipate over 12 to 16 weeks if antipsychotic agents are discontinued" (Kalachnik, Sprague, and Kalies, 1991, p. 3). If stopping the medication is not possible, "an attempt at dose reduction should be considered" (APA Task Force, 1992, p. 237).

Federal Criteria for the Use of Antipsychotic Medication

Because of these risks, HCFA's (1995) Guidance to Surveyors specifies criteria for the use of antipsychotic medications. According to these criteria, antipsychotic medication may be given to a resident (1) who is psychotic, or (2) who has dementia "with associated psychotic and/or agitated behaviors" that are "persistent" and not caused by identifiable triggers (Section F 330, p. 125). The psychosis or behavior must cause a resident to be a danger to self or others; to "continuously scream, yell, or pace if these behaviors cause an impairment in functional capacity;" or to "experience psychotic symptoms" that "cause the resident distress or impairment in functional capacity" (Section F 330, p. 125-126).

After antipsychotic medication is started in an agitated resident with dementia, staff must attempt gradual dose reductions on at least two occasions during the next year, unless the attending physician provides written justification for not doing so. In the case of a resident with psychosis, staff are not *required* to attempt a reduction if the psychotic symptoms "have been stabilized with a maintenance dose of an antipsychotic drug without incurring significant side effects" (HCFA, 1995, Section F 331, p. 127). HCFA (1995) also recommends two annual attempts at reduction for residents taking Benzodiazepines.

As a result of these HCFA guidelines, the use of antipsychotic medication in nursing homes has been reduced by up to 45 percent since the implementation of OBRA 87 (Sakauye, 1995). Studies have shown that when staff are trained to reduce antipsychotic medication for nonpsychotic, nonviolent patients, they can do so for many of them without their demonstrating an increase in behavior problems (Ray et al., 1993; Thapa et al., 1994).

A Caution About Benzodiazepines

While staff are often aware of the serious side effects of antipsychotic medications, they often overlook those for benzodiazepines. Some examples of benzodiazepines are listed under Antianxiety Medications and Sleep Medications in Table 8.1.

There are serious problems with the extended use of benzodiazepines to treat anxiety or agitation, especially in the elderly. They may cause not only sedation and orthostatic hypotension, but also confusional states and impaired memory for recent events (Ashton, 1995). Physical dependence upon benzodiazepines "develops within weeks of regular use" (Miller, 1995, p. 168). When the medication is stopped abruptly, withdrawal symptoms occur in "30 to 45 percent of patients who have used regular therapeutic doses" (Ashton, 1995, p. 163). These symptoms may include anxiety, gastrointestinal upset, depression, headache, seizures, and/or delirium (Miller, 1995).

While benzodiazepines are often given with the intention of calming agitated patients, one risk is that they may cause "paradoxical excitement," manifested by anxiety, insomnia, hyperactivity, and aggressive behavior (Ashton, 1995, p. 160). Similarly, elderly patients taking benzodiazepines for long periods can become more irritable and argumentative, probably because the medications make them less socially inhibited (Ashton, 1995). There is also the possibility that prolonged use of benzodiazepines will "cause or aggravate depression" (Ashton, 1995, p. 161).

Concerning their efficacy, psychiatrist Heather Ashton, DM, notes that benzodiazepines are quite effective for *short-term* treatment of insomnia, "short-term or intermittent treatment of some anxiety disorders," or as a "short-term aid to alcohol/other CNS depressant drug withdrawal" (Ashton, 1995, p. 159). However, she emphasizes that their long-term use is very problematic. When benzodiazepines are used every night to treat insomnia, they lose their efficacy within a few weeks (Ashton, 1995). While patients do experience better sleep initially, they are likely to have returned to their pretreatment levels of delayed sleep onset and of intrasleep awakening within a few weeks (Ashton, 1995). When benzodiazepines are used to treat anxiety, tolerance develops more slowly (Ashton, 1995). However, Dr. Ashton emphasizes that there is little evidence that they "retain their effectiveness after four months of regular treatment, and clinical observations suggest that long-term benzodiazepine use over the years does little to control, and may even aggravate, anxiety states" (1995, p. 161). Consequently, she concludes with the following recommendations about the prescription of benzodiazepines:

> It is recommended that prescriptions should be limited, when possible, to short-term (maximum four weeks) or intermittent courses, in minimal effective doses, and prescribed only when symptoms are severe. Psychological treatments, sometimes combined with antidepressant drugs, are more appropriate in the long term for most patients with anxiety disorders. (Ashton, 1995, p. 164)

Of course, even patients who are prescribed intermittent (PRN) doses of benzodiazepines may end up taking them on a daily basis, either because they request such or because staff decide that the patients need it. Obviously, staff should pay careful attention to how often PRN benzodiazepines are given. If a PRN prescription becomes a daily administration, staff have to evaluate the risks and benefits of such, and consult with the attending physician.

MEDICATION FOR AGITATED RESIDENTS
WITH DEMENTIA

As we mentioned in Chapter 2, agitation is an umbrella term for behaviors like verbal and physical aggression, noisemaking, and wandering. In LTC facilities without psychiatric consultants, medicating agitated residents with dementia presents a very difficult problem for the attending physician and nursing staff. Even psychiatrists are not sure what helps demented residents with agitation. As psychiatrist Kenneth Sakauye, MD, puts it:

> This is a controversial area in which target symptoms are unclear, the mechanism of action (or reason for action) of medications is unclear, and prescribing is still based on clinical judgment without established guidelines. (1995, p. 425)

There are not many well-designed studies of antipsychotic medication with these residents, and those that exist show that it is only slightly effective (Sakauye, 1995). Concerning other kinds of psychiatric medication, there are few good studies that have assessed their efficacy with the demented, agitated elderly (Sakauye, 1995).

However, Sakauye (1995) does offer some guidelines as to when medication for agitation appears appropriate. He states that staff should first look for external causes of the problem and should attempt behavioral interventions. If these efforts fail, he views that failure as one sign that the triggers of the behavior are internal. He also describes three other signs that the causes of the problems are likely internal rather than external: (1) the agitation occurs continuously and at any time of day; (2) the behavior is unplanned, and the resident cannot stop himself; and (3) the resident has a psychiatric diagnosis that accompanies the dementia, such as depression or psychosis. If staff can establish that the agitation fits this pattern, Sakauye believes that they can conclude that the source of the problem is likely internal, making medication a logical choice. Of course, with many residents, a combination of internal and external causes is often at work. In such cases, he believes that internal causes have more influence when "the behaviors are out of proportion to any provocation and are uncontrollable" (Sakauye, 1995, p. 426).

Once staff have ruled out external causes of the agitation and have ruled out psychiatric problems besides dementia, Dr. Sakauye gives the following advice regarding medication:

> Once medication trials are initiated, it is probably best to follow a sequential single therapy approach to try to avoid polypharmacy and the potential negative cognitive effects from drug interactions or high-dose psychotropic medications . . . doses should be low and the patient's status should be monitored frequently.
>
> The initial selection of medication for agitation or depression is, at present, based on clinical judgement. Neuroleptics have been used most frequently. . . . However, our preference has been to use nonneuroleptic management initially unless there are clear psychotic features. Buspirone is one alternative due to its S-1 serotonergic activity and low sedation and side effect profile. The usual starting dose is 5 mg tid, increased rapidly until behavioral improvement is noted or the maximum dose of 60 mg per day is reached. Alternatively, trazodone HCI is often used, especially if there is a need for sedation or presence of dysphoric mood. Doses of 50 mg per day are usually sufficient for behavioral improvement. However, concomitant neuroleptic medications may be required for acute behavioral problems at the beginning of a trial.
>
> After four weeks at maximum doses, a medication change is considered if there has been minimal improvement in target symptoms. If there has been no significant improvement throughout the initial medication trial, we usually substitute a neuroleptic if it has not been tried initially. If a neuroleptic has failed or is not tolerated, we generally will seek a different nonneuroleptic medication described above or an SSRI (Selective Serotonin Reuptake Inhibitor) if there is mild dysphoric mood without a need for sedation.
>
> . . . . Benzodiazepines are rarely used due to our experience of excessive sedation, confusion, and gait disturbance at therapeutic doses for this frail population . . . .
>
> . . . . Throughout medication trials, attempts are made to help the staff develop behavioral treatment approaches, especially around communication skills and low-stimulus environments in

an attempt to reduce potential environmental factors that might escalate pathological behavior. (Sakauye, 1995, pp. 429-430; reproduced by permission of SLACK, Inc.)

In a personal communication on April 1, 1996, Dr. Sakauye cautioned that not all psychiatrists would agree with him, as some would prefer to use antipsychotic medications first. He also said that the efficacy of buspirone with agitated, demented patients is currently being tested via a national multisite study. Its results should be available by the time this book is published.

THE PSYCHOTROPIC MEDICATION COMMITTEE

As you can see from the preceding discussion, using psychiatric medication in LTC is a difficult, risky, and complicated undertaking. Without a clear consensus from the psychiatric community on how agitation should be medicated, staff must pool their training, clinical skills, and observations to arrive at optimal decisions.

For this reason, having a multidisciplinary psychotropic medication committee in each LTC facility is ideal. The purpose of the committee is to review the treatment of residents taking psychoactive medications and to make recommendations. The committee can help the facility meet OBRA's requirements for reducing medications, for scheduling medication holidays, and for using these medications only to treat a diagnosed problem. In addition, the committee can help staff comply with federal regulations, such as those for antipsychotic drugs discussed above. Often, these criteria are not met in LTC because residents are admitted with psychotropic prescriptions, staff are not trained to develop behavioral interventions, and staff call the attending physician about a problem only when it becomes intolerable, leading to a quick decision to medicate.

The psychotropic medication committee should include a number of disciplines. A registered nurse, who is familiar with the cases under discussion, should attend. A staff member from the medical records department can take notes and communicate the committee's recommendations to the charge nurses and attending physician. A pharmacist may provide information to the committee about medication interactions, specific medications to address a given problem, titration and dosages, and regulations related to psychotropic medications. The social services designee provides an overview of the problem, including psychosocial causes of the problem and behavioral interventions that have been attempted. The social services consultant and mental health consultant can also be quite helpful, especially when they are familiar with the residents under discussion. In some facilities, the medical director, administrator, DON, LVNs, or NAs participate in this committee.

Each month, the committee reviews residents taking psychoactive medications, and writes a brief report on each for the attending physician. The committee discusses and reports on the following aspects of each resident's care: psychotropic medications, dosages, and frequency; psychiatric diagnosis; behavior(s) exhibited; summary of adverse side effects, if any, over the last month; psychosocial and behavioral interventions used; whether the behavior is worse, the same, or better; and recommendations about medications and psychosocial interventions. The committee's recommendations may be to reduce or discontinue the medication, try an alternative medication, use drug holidays, and/or attempt different behavioral approaches. Table 8.3 provides an example of a report from psychotropic medication committee.

The committee's reports are not usually placed in the medical record, but in a binder maintained by the committee. However, its findings and recommendations should be recorded in the nursing or social services notes, and corresponding adjustments to the care plan should be made.

Once the committee has completed its reports, staff communicate their recommendations to the physician. In some facilities, the DON or a charge nurse calls the attending physician or sends him the summary. In others, a charge nurse gives him a copy at the next on-site visit.

Finally, minutes of the committee's meetings are taken by one of the attending staff members, usually the person from the medical records department. The minutes provide a listing of the residents discussed and a one- or two-line synopsis of the committee's recommendations for each. The committee members review the minutes at the next meeting and initial their approval. These minutes are then placed in the binder maintained by the committee.

TABLE 8.3. Example of a Report from a Psychotropic Medication Committee

Date: _____

1. Medication, dose, and frequency: *Buspar 10 mg TID*

2. Diagnosis: *Alzheimer's Dementia*

3. Behavior exhibited: *resists care, strikes out at staff, visual hallucinations.*

4. Adverse medication reactions (circle): sedation, anticholinergic
(describe _____).
extrapyramidal (describe _____).
orthostatic hypotension, constipation, hypertension, ataxia, tachycardia, dystonias, other: *none.*
If resident is taking an antipsychotic medication, date and score of most recent assessment for Tardive Dyskinesia: *DISCUS score of 0 on June 2, 1996.*

5. Psychosocial and behavioral interventions used: *Staff approach her slowly from the front to avoid startling her. During ADLs, staff leave if she resists or hits and try again later. Staff praise cooperation during ADLs.*

6. Evaluation: _____x_____ behavior(s) have not changed
_____ behavior(s) have improved
_____ behavior(s) have worsened

7. Recommendations: *Recommend .5 mg Risperdal for visual hallucinations. Haldol is not recommended due to her previous bad reaction. Continue Buspar, but reduce if sedation occurs. CNA will ambulate her twice a day.*

Signatures

Resident's name: _____ Room _____

Attending Physician: _____

CONCLUSION

Hopefully, over the next few years, studies will offer solid evidence about which medications are helpful in controlling agitation in elderly residents with dementia. We also hope that consultation from geropsychiatrists will be more readily available to attending physicians and nursing staff. Even then, however, there will be a place for the expertise and vigilance provided by a multidisciplinary psychotropic medication committee. Such a committee can not only help staff to arrive at better decisions regarding medications, but can also to meet the ever-increasing requirements for documentation in LTC. Effective documentation is topic of our next chapter.

REFERENCES

American Psychiatric Association Task Force on Tardive Dyskinesia (1992). *Tardive dyskinesia: A task force report of the American Psychiatric Association.* Washington, DC: American Psychiatric Association.

Ashton, H. (1995). Toxicity and adverse consequences of benzodiasepine use. *Psychiatric Annals, 25*, 158-165.

Bezchlibnyk-Butler, K.Z., Jeffries, J.J., and Martin, B.A. (1994). *Clinical handbook of psychotropic drugs.* Seattle: Hogrefe and Huber.

Cole, J.O. and Yonkers, K.A. (1995). Nonbenzodiazepine anxiolytics. In A.F. Schatzberg and C.B. Nemeroff (Eds.), *The American psychiatric press textbook of psychopharmacology.* Washington, DC: American Psychiatric Press.

Ereshefsky, L. (1995). Treatment strategies for schizophrenia. *Psychiatric Annals,* 25, 285-296.

Health Care Financing Administration (1995). *State operations manual: Provider certification.* Washington, DC: Health Care Finance Administration. (National Technical Information Source No. PB 95950009.)

Hermann, N. (1992). Principles of geriatric psychopharmacology. In D.K. Conn, N. Hermann, A. Kaye, D. Rewilak, A. Robinson, and B. Schogt (Eds.), *Practical psychiatry in the nursing home* (pp. 177-191). Seattle: Hogrefe and Huber.

Kalachnik, J.E., Sprague, R.L., and Kalies, R. (1991). *Tardive dyskinesia monitoring and the DISCUS* [manual and videotaped training program]. East Hanover, NJ: Sandoz Pharmaceuticals. (Available from Sandoz Pharmaceuticals, 59 Rt. 10, E. Hanover, NJ 07936.)

Mendelowitz, A.J. and Lieberman, J.A. (1995). New findings in the use of atypical antipsychotic drugs: I: Focus on risperidone. *The Journal of Clinical Psychiatry Case and Comment Series, 2:1*, 1-12.

Miller, N.S. (1995). Liability and efficacy from long-term use of benzodiazepines: Documentation and interpretation. *Psychiatric Annals, 25*, 166-172.

Neylan, T.C., De May, M.D., and Reynolds, C.F. (1996). Sleep and chronobiological disturbances. In E.W. Busse and D.G. Blazer (Eds.), *The American psychiatric press textbook of geriatric psychiatry,* 2nd Edition, (pp. 329-340). Washington, DC: American Psychiatric Press.

Ray, W.A., Taylor, J.A., Meador, K.G., Lichtenstein, M.J., Griffin, M.R., Fought, R., Adams, M.L., and Blazer, D.G. (1993). Reducing antipsychotic drug use in nursing homes. *Archives of Internal Medicine, 153,* 713-721.

Sakauye, K. (1995). Behavioral disturbances: Pharmacologic therapies. *Psychiatric Annals, 25,* 425-431.

Salzman, C., Satlin, A., and Burrows, A.B. (1995). Geriatric psychopharmacology. In A.F. Schatzberg and C.B. Nemeroff (Eds.), *The American Psychiatric Press textbook of psychopharmacology* (pp. 803-816). Washington, DC: American Psychiatric Press.

Stoudemire, A., Moran, M.D., and Fogel, B.S. (1995). Psychopharmacology in the medically ill patient. In A.F. Schatzberg and C. Nemeroff (Eds.), *The American Psychiatric Press textbook of psychopharmacology.* Washington, DC: American Psychiatric Press.

Thapa, P.B., Meador, K.G., Gideon, P., Fought, R., and Ray, W.A. (1994). Effects of antipsychotic withdrawal in elderly nursing home residents. *Journal of the American Geriatrics Society, 42,* 280-286.

Wise, M.G., and Rundell, J.R. (1995). *Consultation psychiatry,* second edition. Washington, DC: American Psychiatric Press.

Chapter 9

Administrative Issues:
The Resident Assessment Instrument (RAI)
and Preparation for Survey

Perhaps the most cumbersome part of working in LTC is the extensive documentation required of staff. Most people choose helping professions in order to make a difference in the lives of others. When paperwork overwhelms their opportunities for intervening with patients, work becomes more tedious and less meaningful.

In this chapter, our aim is to help you "work smart, not hard" when it comes to these administrative demands. First, we provide a basic overview of the Resident Assessment Instrument (RAI). In the following section, we describe the survey process and highlight common deficiencies cited by surveyors. We close with a brief description of the nursing home as a family system and how that can impact the survey process. In addition, please refer to the appedixes for additional resource information related to these issues.

THE RESIDENT ASSESSMENT INSTRUMENT (RAI)

Providing quality care for LTC residents begins with gathering information. How well a resident is treated is largely determined by how effectively staff assess the resident and share the results among themselves and with the attending physician. The purpose of the Resident Assessment Instrument (RAI), mandated by OBRA 87, is to optimize this process. Specifically, it provides a framework for staff's assessing residents, communicating the results, and making clinical decisions.

The original impetus for the RAI came from the Institute of Medicine's 1986 report, which recommended (1) that each resident should have a comprehensive assessment and treatment plan, (2) that this plan should be applied in a coordinated way, and (3) that a resident assessment package should be created for facilities certified by Medicare and Medicaid.

Consequently, in 1990, the HCFA published the original RAI, which consisted of the Minimum Data Set (MDS) or Minimum Data Set Plus (MDS+), triggers, Resident Assessment Protocols (RAPs), and the official Utilization Guidelines. By 1991, all states were using the RAI. Later, HCFA revised the MDS, creating the MDS 2.0, which was implemented on January 1, 1996. From HCFA's standpoint, the advantages of having a national assessment tool are that (1) data on patient care can be transmitted electronically and monitored for quality and compliance purposes, and (2) data can be used for research and policy analysis.

In describing the assessment process and its documentation, we will follow a sequence of steps, as shown in Figure 9.1. All of these fall under the umbrella of the RAI.

FIGURE 9.1. Key Steps in the Assessment Process

MDS 2.0 ⟶ Triggers ⟶ RAPS ⟶

RAP Summary Sheet ⟶ Care Plan ⟶ Documentation

The Minimum Data Set 2.0 (MDS 2.0)

The MDS 2.0 is a screening instrument providing the "minimum" assessment required. The most psychosocially relevant sections are E, "Mood and Behavior Patterns"; and F, "Psychosocial Well-being." Other relevant sections are B, "Cognitive Patterns"; C, "Communication/Hearing Patterns"; and Q, "Discharge Potential and Overall Status."

To illustrate the format and content of the MDS 2.0, Section F, psychosocial Well-being, is reproduced in Table 9.1. The items assess how well the resident has adjusted to the nursing home, and staff check those that are true of the resident. For example, item three asks about

TABLE 9.1. Section F (Psychosocial Well-Being) of the MDS 2.0

1. Sense of Initiative/Involvement

At ease interacting with others — a. _____
At ease doing planned or structured activities — b. _____
At ease doing self-initiated activities — c. _____
Establishes own goals — d. _____
Pursues involvement in life of facility (e.g., makes/keeps friends; involved in group activities; responds positively to new activities; assists at religious services) — e. _____
Accepts invitations into most group activities — f. _____
NONE OF THE ABOVE — g. _____

2. Unsettled Relationships

Covert/open conflict with or repeated criticism of staff — a. _____
Unhappy with roommate — b. _____
Unhappy with residents other than roommate — c. _____
Openly expresses conflict/anger with family/friends — d. _____
Absence of personal contact with family/friends — e. _____
Recent loss of close family member/friend — f. _____
Does not adjust easily to change in routines — g. _____
NONE OF THE ABOVE — h. _____

3. Past Roles

Strong identification with past roles and life status — a. _____
Expresses sadness/anger/empty feeling over lost roles/status — b. _____
Resident perceives that daily routine (customary routine, activities) is very different from prior pattern in the community — c. _____
NONE OF THE ABOVE — d. _____

Source: HCFA, October, 1995.

153

the resident's perception of his current role and routine, as compared with previous roles and routines.

In Section E, "Mood and Behavior Patterns," two scales are used to quantify "Behavioral Symptoms": one for the "frequency" of the problem and one for the "alterability" of the behavior over the last seven days. To complete these items, you can draw on staff's hash-mark tracking or analyze data from a tracking grid like that presented in Figure 6.5 in Chapter 6.

Section P, "Special Treatment and Procedures," is a new section in the MDS 2.0. Here, staff record adjunctive treatments that the resident has received, including psychosocial ones such as psychotherapy, behavioral assessments, and environmental changes.

Triggers

Because the MDS 2.0 is a screening tool and not an in-depth assessment, it provides staff with criteria for deciding when a resident needs a detailed evaluation in certain areas. These criteria are provided in the form of "triggers," which are noted in each section of the MDS 2.0. These sections correspond to a specific "Resident Assessment Protocol" (RAP) that needs to "worked" when triggered. For example, certain scores in the "Behavioral Symptoms" section trigger the Behavior Problems RAP. The 18 RAPs in the MDS 2.0 are shown in Table 9.2.

Resident Assessment Protocols (RAPs)

RAPs guidelines require that in doing an in-depth evaluation, staff must describe the following:

- The nature of the problem, as portrayed by the resident's subjective complaints and objective data (e.g., the number of times per week it has occurred).
- "Complications and risk factors that affect the decision to proceed to care planning."
- Which aspects of the problem, if any, you will incorporate into the care plan.
- Whether there is a need for further evaluation by the appropriate health care professional.

TABLE 9.2. The 18 Resident Assessment Protocols

1. Delirium
2. Cognitive Loss
3. Visual Function
4. Communication
5. ADL functional/rehabilitation potential
6. Urinary incontinence and indwelling catheter
7. Psychosocial well-being
8. Mood state
9. Behavioral symptoms
10. Activities
11. Falls
12. Nutritional status
13. Feeding tubes
14. Dehydration/fluid maintenance
15. Dental care
16. Pressure ulcers
17. Psychotropic drug use
18. Physical restraints

Source: HFCA, October, 1995.

For example, for the Behavior Symptoms, RAP staff must describe factors such as (1) the behavior itself, including possible triggers related to time and place; (2) whether psychiatric or medical diagnoses are possible causes of the problem; (3) whether there is need for evaluation by a professional; and (4) a statement justifying staff's decision to include the problem in the care plan or not (HCFA, October, 1995).

Unlike the MDS 2.0, for which there is a standard HCFA form, there is no form for the RAPs. Each facility may create its own form, or may document RAPs information throughout the medical record in areas such as progress notes, mental health evaluations, flow sheets, or RAP modules. Like the MDS 2.0, most RAPs forms are easy to follow and self-explanatory.

Now let's look at an example of the RAPs process using the Mood State section of the MDS 2.0. A staff member notes that a new resident has periods of crying (MDS item E-1m), self-deprecating remarks (MDS item E-1e), and withdrawal from activities of interest (MDS item E-1o). She also notes that efforts to console or reassure the resident (MDS item E-2) are relatively ineffective. These results trigger the Mood RAP. Following the guidelines in HCFA's October 1995 manual, the staff member investigates a number of contributing factors, including history, delirium, recent losses, change in body image, diagnoses, and medication. She also notes sections cross-referenced in the MDS 2.0, and then arrives at an accurate assessment. This then leads to the RAP Summary (Section V).

RAP Summary (MDS 2.0, Section V)

In the Summary section of the MDS 2.0, the staff member checks off the RAP problem areas that have been triggered; the location and date of the RAP documentation; and whether, given the results of the RAP, "a new care plan, care plan revision, or continuation of current care plan is necessary." In the case of the depressed resident, the staff member notes that his documentation is located on a given date in the Social Services progress notes. He also documents that a referral has been made to the mental health consultant. He then works on the care plan.

The Interdisciplinary Resident Care Plan

Comprehensive care plans are mandated by HCFA (June, 1995), as indicated by the following excerpt:

> The facility must develop a comprehensive care plan for each resident that includes measurable objectives and timetables to meet a resident's medical, nursing, and psychosocial needs, that are identified in the comprehensive assessment. A comprehensive care plan must be developed within seven days after completion of the comprehensive assessment . . . and prepared by an interdisciplinary team. (HCFA, June 1995, pp. 77-78)

The care plan is the specific plan of action for a particular resident. The plan defines the resident's unique problems and focuses upon goals that are realistic and measurable. As goals are met and new needs arise, the care plan is revised, and it must be reviewed at least every 90 days at care-planning conferences.

In the case of the depressed resident described above, the staff member could now use several sources of information in forming the care plan: the initial social services and nursing assessments, the MDS 2.0, the RAPs, feedback from staff and family, and perhaps data from behavioral tracking. Once this "homework" is complete, writing the care plan is relatively easy.

The care plan itself describes the problem, the goal, and the interventions used to achieve the goal. We now discuss each of these parts.

The Problem

The first column of the care plan asks for a specific, behaviorally stated problem. You can use the terminology of the MDS 2.0 if you wish. The most important point is that you include a specific description of the how the problem is manifested. Returning to our example, if the physician or mental health consultant had made a diagnosis of depression, then you could state the problem as follows: "Depression manifested by periods of tearfulness, self-deprecating statements, and withdrawal or self-isolation."

The Goal

The goal should address the problem directly, should be realistic and measurable, and should include a time frame. To meet these criteria, you can ask yourself three questions as you write goals:

- What do I want to see change?
- How can I measure the change?
- When might this change have occurred?

Returning to our depressed resident, the staff member wants the resident to be less depressed. How would he measure this? There are a number of ways, but here is one possibility: "She will display only one period of tearfulness per week; she will make one positive statement about herself each week during counseling; and she will attend one activity per week." These would be especially good goals if staff had been recording their frequency prior to intervening with her depression. In this way, the staff member would know how frequently these behaviors were occurring, and thus could establish realistic short-term goals. These goals should be evaluated every 90 days and, if necessary, revised.

The Approaches

The "Approach" is the intervention that the interdisciplinary team uses to attain the goals. In the case of our depressed resident, these might include the following: weekly counseling sessions with the social worker, encouragement to attend activities, and visitation by family members during mealtime to make eating a more pleasant activity. If she was taking an antidepressant, it would be listed after these psychosocial interventions, in order lend more emphasis to the behavioral approaches. Such is even more important when the resident is taking an antipsychotic or antianxiety medication.

Once the care plan is completed, staff must implement it. Staff must carry out the intervention, monitor the results, and revise the care plan on a quarterly basis. Quantitative monitoring of the behavior is absolutely essential. In the case of our depressed resident, we would track the frequency of her crying, self-deprecating remarks, and participation in activities. Such would provide a behavioral barometer of the effectiveness of the counseling, medication, and staff's encouragement to participate in activities.

In this book, we do not describe in detail the design and implementation of care plans. There are a number of excellent books on care planning that we recommend, several of which are listed in Appendix A. The care plan samples in these books are particularly helpful.

Documentation

Once the RAPs and care plan are complete, staff must document their ongoing implementation of the care plan. For the social services department, a quarterly summary must be provided on each resident. Residents with psychosocial problems need more frequent documentation from social services staff. For a summary of areas to cover in the quarterly progress notes, see Table 9.3.

TABLE 9.3. Recommended Content for Social Services' Quarterly Progress Notes

- Brief summary of mental and physical status
- Changes in mental or physical status
- Whether resident needs assistance with ADLs or ambulation
- Whether resident is incontinent or continent
- Nutrition, e.g., weight changes and assistance for eating.
- Management of personal and financial affairs
- Visitors and their frequency of visitation
- Activities and how often the resident participates
- Potential for alternative placement
- Interventions for meeting care plan goals, and their impact
- List additions or deletions to care plan
- Special needs addressed, e.g., glasses, clothing

We recommend that if social services staff have access to a computer, they use word processing for the quarterly notes. Once the first note is completed, staff can use it as the basis for the next quarterly report.

SURVEY ISSUES

Perhaps nothing stresses LTC staff more than a visit from the state surveyor. One key to minimizing the stress involved is to be constantly prepared for a survey. In this section, we describe guidelines for being "survey-ready," provide you with a summary of the forms and criteria used by surveyors, and summarize the common deficiencies cited by surveyors at our LTC facilities. Because most of our work in this area has been with the social services staff, much of our specific discussion will focus upon how they would prepare for a survey. However, nurses should also benefit from our more general discussion of the guidelines and common deficiencies.

Guidelines for Being "Survey-Ready"

Understand the survey process. If you understand what a survey involves, your preparation will be easier and much more effective.

What observations and inspections will surveyors make? What questions will they ask, and of whom? To answer these questions, we have provided you with a summary of the following HCFA forms and guidelines: HCFA's requirements for the social services department (Appendix B), surveyors' individual and group interview questions (Appendix C), surveyors' observations of noninterviewable residents (Appendix D), surveyors' family interview questions (Appendix E), surveyors' resident review worksheet (Appendix F), and surveyors' general observations of a facility (Appendix G). You can use these Appendixes, or the actual HCFA forms on which they are based, to do mock surveys (see below).

Know the regulations. The most important psychosocially-related regulations concern residents' rights and quality of life. To become thoroughly familiar with these, review sections from the Guidance to Surveyors HCFA (in June, 1995) entitled Social Services (483.15), Resident Rights (483.10 and 483.12), and Quality of Life (483.15).

Since surveyors ask patients if they have been informed of their rights and know them, you should constantly educate your residents about them. There are a number of ways to do this. As a survey date approaches, you can review rights with your alert and oriented residents at the resident council. Some facilities use a "Residents' Right of the Week," which is posted in the activities room and reviewed throughout the week prior to an activity. There is also a commercially available bingo game for teaching residents their rights.

Review the OSCAR. The Online Survey Certification and Reporting System (OSCAR) is HCFA's computerized means of providing current information about survey results. Through it, users can readily access the survey results for all LTC facilities that are Medicare or Medicaid providers. By accessing the OSCAR you can obtain a summary of your facility's deficiencies over the previous four years. In this way, you can make sure that past problems have been corrected. In the current survey process, there is little tolerance for repeated deficiencies.

Know your residents. While knowing your residents sounds like an obvious requirement, it is surprising how often staff do not know all of their residents' needs. The key to knowing your residents is to do a thorough initial assessment and careful ongoing assessments during your one-to-one visits. Even when surveyors examine the outcome of staff's interventions, they always trace them back through the implementation process to the original evaluation. In the process of doing assessments, social services staff should develop a "critical list" of residents with prominent psychosocial issues. This list comprises the 20 percent of all residents who consume 80 percent of the social worker's time. To stay abreast of residents' needs, you should write quarterly notes on all of them and more frequent notes on the 20 percent with special needs. While doing your assessments, ask yourself what a resident might tell a surveyor about her needs, preferences, and quality of life in the facility.

Use your Quality Assurance (QA) Program. Most facilities have a QA program, which is designed to identify and correct problems with assessment and treatment. Whether your QA program uses traditional QA tools, Total Quality Management (TQM), or Continuous Quality Improvement (CQI), use the process as a "mini survey" to identify and correct problem areas that might be flagged by a surveyor.

Have a mock survey. Your social services consultant or a sister facility could do this for you. Mock surveys may include the use of probes (questions that the surveyors ask residents), the administration of resident satisfaction questionnaires, a review of prior survey findings, an evaluation of documentation, a review of the theft and loss program, an evaluation of staff's follow-up on residents' grievances, and an overall look at a department's compliance with regulations.

Use your time wisely. Time management is critical for your survival in LTC, especially in preparing for survey. As survey draws near, make a prioritized list of what you need to do to prepare for it. To manage your time efficiently, use some of the suggestions we give you at the end of Chapter 11.

The Survey Itself: Some Guidelines

When the survey team arrives, many facilities use a standard alert code, announced over the intercom, to inform staff of its arrival. The alert code may consist of a message such as "Dr. Quintero, a call for you on line two."

When answering questions from the survey team, answer only the questions asked; do not volunteer information. If you are not sure of an answer, say so, and then find out and communicate the answer as soon as possible. Have information at your fingertips, including your policies and procedures manuals, grievance logs, resident council minutes, and theft-and-loss logs. Above all, have key information and documentation about your residents readily available, if not in your head.

We have included Appendix H, which summarizes what the survey team wants within 24 hours of entering. Of particular interest to social workers are #4 discharges, #9 hospice patients, #10 dialysis patients, #11 residents under age 55, and #12 residents with potential communication problems.

Following Survey

Following a survey, staff are given a summary of the survey results at the exit conference. These are later followed by the infamous Form 2567, which notes the specific deficiencies and their corresponding regulations. It also includes a summary of the deficiencies in the form of a Scope and Severity Grid (Appendix I).

A Plan of Correction is then required. This plan shows that the facility has corrected the deficiencies and how it plans to prevent the problems from recurring. Staff who have never seen a Plan of Correction can look at those for former surveys. By law, the last one must be posted for review.

In outlining your Plan of Correction, you can address deficiencies by asking yourself the following questions:

- What corrective actions will be taken for residents affected by the deficient practice?
- How will you identify other residents who are at risk for the same deficient practice, and how will you prevent them from experiencing the deficient practice?
- What systematic changes will you make to ensure that the deficient practice does not recur?
- How will you assess whether these systematic changes are working?

Your Quality Assurance program can be one means of addressing these issues. In addition, your Social Services or Nurse Consultant can help you to answer these questions and to monitor ongoing compliance with your plan.

Specific Areas of Deficiency in Surveys

In this section, we summarize the social services-related deficiencies that surveyors cited over a six-year period in five northern California districts.

Documentation of Intervention. This was the most frequently cited area. This area focuses on the following question: what are the resident's needs and problems, and what have staff done about them? Specific issues ranged from concrete needs, such as hearing/vision, clothing, and transportation, to broader psychosocial needs, such as those triggered by the MDS in the areas of mood and behavior problems. With regard to these broader needs, the essential issue is whether staff had a plan for addressing the need and carried it out, not whether staff solved the problem. The problems themselves should be described in the care plan and the interventions documented in the progress notes. If you have stated in the chart that you are planning to do an intervention, such as calling someone, there must be documentation that you followed through.

Continuity. Do the MDS, RAPs, care plan, and progress notes flow logically from one to the other? Were assessments accurate, thorough, timely, and signed?

Care Plans. Surveyors frequently flag care plans that are not revised periodically, especially when a problem persists. They also object to care plans that lump together mood and behavioral problems without providing specific, measurable goals.

Social services staff should keep in mind that their scope of care planning involves more than problems related to mood and behavior. They should provide help with other problem areas, such as cognition, hearing/vision problems, restraints, and perhaps dietary issues. In particular, social services staff should be involved in evaluating the necessity of physical restraints. While residents are usually restrained for their own safety, they may experience anxiety, boredom, depression, and frustration when restrained. For these reasons, staff should make every effort to use the least restrictive measures to ensure patient safety, and they should document their attempts to do so.

Grievances. All grievances from individuals, the resident council, or the family council should generate a plan of correction or documentation of the problem's resolution. The social services staff must usually follow up on the plan of action, ensure that the problem is resolved, and in some cases, have the administrator sign off on the documentation. For both grievances and theft-and-loss incidents, staff should follow their facility's procedures to the letter.

Repeat Survey Issues. Review the OSCAR to ascertain that previous deficiencies have been corrected. There must be a plan in place to ensure compliance with the particular regulation.

Psychotropic Medication. Wherever possible, behavioral interventions should be attempted prior to starting psychotropic medication. For those taking psychiatric medication, behavioral interventions should also be in place. Staff should make sure that a psychiatric diagnosis is the reason for the medication prescription, should use the least restrictive medication, should use drug holidays where possible, and should note attempts to reduce medication. A psychotropic medication committee, described in the Chapter 8, is invaluable in helping staff to implement these guidelines.

Residents' Special Needs. Surveyors often criticize social services staff for their failure to address the psychosocial needs of certain types of residents, such as the terminally ill, those under age 55, the developmentally disabled, and inappropriately placed residents. For the terminally ill, was there a referral to hospice or the clergy? Did staff place younger residents in touch with community resources? Did staff coordinate care for the developmentally disabled with the state agencies serving them? For inappropriately placed residents, such as those who wander into others' rooms or are physically abusive, have staff explored a possible transfer or attempted other means of addressing the residents' problems?

Discharge Planning. This has become an increasingly sensitive area because of managed care, budget cuts, and Medicaid reimbursement. The initial discharge plan should say why the resident needs a SNF and what plans the resident and family have made for meeting this need. If the process proceeds to an actual discharge, social services staff should coordinate follow-up care, complete their portion of the post-discharge plan of care, and provide follow-up in compliance with their state or company regulations. In the case of involuntary discharges, staff must follow the guidelines described in the "Discharge and Transfer" section of Guidance to Surveyors (HCFA, June, 1995). A 30-day notice must be issued and all issues related to the discharge must be documented in detail. Residents are entitled to a fair hearing, which can result in denial of the discharge.

Medicare and Medicaid. Facilities are sometimes cited for failing to provide information about benefits under Medicare and Medicaid. We suggest that you post information on the consumer board. Social services staff should be knowledgable about the application process and the criteria for eligibility, and should be available to consult with families about the application process.

Mental Health Coordination. When patients are evaluated and followed by mental health consultants, your progress notes should describe how you are coordinating the mental health care. You should also note the consultants' findings, recommendations, and medication changes. You can incorporate some of these into your care plans.

Confidentiality. LTC facilities are quite vulnerable in this area. Staff should ensure confidentiality when discussing resident care. They should make sure that no information about residents' problems is posted in rooms or other public areas.

Resident Abuse. Preventing abuse is the first mandate of both the Department of Health and the ombudsman. As "in-house" advocates for residents, staff should evaluate allegations of abuse, follow state-mandated procedures for reporting, counsel residents, and take steps to prevent reoccurrences.

Family Intervention. Some family-related problems require intervention and referral to community resources. For example, a resident's relative may need psychotherapy or financial or legal assistance. Where family members are interfering with the resident's care, staff can request evaluation and intervention from their mental health consultant, and they should document their interventions in the care plan and progress notes. Since there is often not sufficient time to hear all of the family's concerns during the quarterly care planning conference, social services staff may need to schedule an appointment with them after the conference. Social services staff usually coordinate the family council and follow up on grievances or problems that they raise. Their work with the family council should be clearly documented.

Residents of Foreign Nationality. Residents who speak a foreign language must have a care plan that addresses this barrier to communication. The care plan should state how the resident will communicate with staff. While interpreters are always desirable, communication boards or cards can be used. Documentation in the chart must indicate that they have received a copy of all important documents in their own language, including residents' rights, advance directives material, house rules, residents' responsibilities, informed consents, and admission agreements. In lieu of having these translated into the resident's language, it is sufficient to document that a family member or interpreter has explained these to the resident.

Conflicting Documentation. Such is likely to occur if assessments are not accurate and the interdisciplinary team is not communicating. Staff should read the notes of those from other disciplines prior to writing their own progress notes. If discrepancies in assessment or observation occur, clarify them in the IDT meeting prior to making progress notes.

Body Image. Staff frequently overlook how residents feel about their physical problems and losses, and about the resulting change in their body image. These physical problems and losses may include a recent colostomy, amputation, CVA with altered bodily functions, chemotherapy with hair loss, or uncontrollable motor functions. Staff should document how residents have reacted to these changes and what interventions have been provided.

Room Changes. State surveyors try to determine if room changes are made for the sake of staff's needs rather than residents' needs. They give deficiencies for frequent or unnecessary room changes for which there is not sufficient explanation. HCFA guidelines emphasize that room changes must follow specific guidelines. All residents affected must agree and receive notification of the change. The rationale for every room change must be documented. A facility can never change a patient's room for the sake of monetary gain.

Residents' Self-Determination. While surveyors do evaluate this area, it is one frequently overlooked by staff. All alert and oriented residents should be involved in their care planning and in the signing of the following documents: the advance directives, residents' rights, informed consents, and admissions agreement. If the resident is incapable of participating in these ways, such must be indicated in writing by the physician or the mental health consultant. In borderline cases in which the resident displays minor or fluctuating cognitive impairment, both the resident and the responsible party can sign the documents and participate in care planning.

Consumer Board. HCFA guidelines mandate that residents have access to certain information. The most important piece of information is the most recent facility survey. One way to make this accessible to residents is to have it laminated, placed in a binder, attached to the wall by a chain, and held by a plastic wall receptacle. The chain and lamination ensure that confused residents will not take it away or damage it. Information that can be placed on a bulletin board includes the following: the ombudsman's name, address, and phone number; a large print edition of residents' rights; mental health advocacy agencies; eligibility information about Medicare and Medicaid; the agency to which Medicaid fraud can be reported; local centers for the developmentally disabled; and a statement indicating how complaints can be filed with the Department of Health. While it is not mandatory, we recommend that you also post the grievance policy with blank forms, the policy regarding privacy of phone use, voting procedures, theft-and-loss policy, and social services referral forms and procedures.

Sound Levels. Staff have been written up for being too loud or permitting residents to be too noisy. Surveyors have cited disturbing intercom systems, loud pill-crushing devices, and screaming residents who disturb others.

Residents' Rights. The Department of Health repeatedly focuses upon the facility's responsibility to protect and promote the rights of residents by informing them of these rights at admission and throughout the course of their stay. Surveyors focus on the following rights: the use of interest-bearing accounts (trusts) and the accessibility of funds on weekends, the ability of residents to exercise their right to vote, communication of rights in the resident's own language, and whether intramuscular psychiatric medications are given without consent to residents who do not have a conservatorship with court-granted permission to receive such medications. In addition, surveyors evaluate whether there is a home-like environment, as manifested by the availability of chairs for visitors and the presence of wall decor and furnishings. They also want to know if mail is delivered promptly, including on weekends. Finally, they notice whether staff respect residents' rights in more subtle ways. For example, do staff walk through the activity room when an activity is in progress?

Right to Inspect and Photocopy Charts. Not only should staff inform residents of their rights in this regard, they should inform them about problems that are being addressed by staff. At times, rapport between residents and staff is damaged when residents read their charts and are surprised to find problems documented that were never discussed with them.

Privacy. Staff should ensure that privacy curtains are used. For cognitively intact residents, staff should knock on the door and wait for a response before entering. If student trainees come to the facility to see specific residents, permission should be obtained from these residents.

Terminology. Surveyors cite language that is inappropriate, unprofessional, or derogatory. The following are examples that have been cited: use of "patients" rather than "residents" (unless they are in a subacute or rehab facility); use of "feeder" instead of "assisted dining"; use of "chronic complainer" instead of "voicing multiple concerns"; using judgmental terms such as "sloppy," "bossy," and "whining"; and using substitutes for names, such as "honey" and "sweetie".

Pets. While pets may have benefits for the elderly, facilities have been written up for failing to safeguard against health hazards. The facility should maintain records of veterinary care, shots, veterinarian phone numbers, and cleaning and feeding schedules. Staff should also remember that the cleaning of cages and litter boxes is an infection control issue.

THE NURSING HOME "FAMILY" AND THE SURVEY PROCESS

Thus far, we have discussed only the content of the survey and what you as an individual or team can do to prepare for such. Obviously, however, you are participating in a larger nursing home organization that operates as a "family." The "family members" have ways of treating and communicating with each other that enhance or hinder their preparation for survey, the impression left with the surveyor, and the quality of treatment given to residents. These ways of treating and communicating with one another are *process* issues rather than *content* issues. Destructive processes within the nursing home family can override even the most conscientious efforts of individuals and teams.

Types of Nursing Home Families

In our experience, there are at least three types of nursing home "families": the nurturing type, the inadequate type, and the destructive type. Many homes are combinations of these.

A nurturing nursing home family maintains open communication, takes a democratic approach to management, and acknowledges the contributions of its staff. Staff members freely approach managers about problems, feel that their issues are heard, and can propose ideas that managers will consider in developing a solution. Managers also communicate clearly and consistently what is expected from their employees. They acknowledge compliance and appropriately confront those who fall short. When conflicts arise among team members, management intervenes early in the process. If a resolution cannot be reached, action is taken so that the destructive relationships do not fester.

In an inadequate nursing home, family managers are apathetic or detached. Staff members do not believe managers are interested in hearing about problems or their ideas for solving them. Managers give the message: "I don't want to hear about another problem." They do not make clear what is expected of their employees, though they may criticize employees later on for failing to do what they never asked them to do in the first place. Good work is rarely noticed and never praised. Conflicts among team members are allowed to fester until they are out of control. In sum, the inadequate nursing home family hurts itself through management that is too passive.

By contrast, in a destructive nursing home family, there is open conflict, frequent backstabbing, and aggressive criticism. Managers are authoritarian and reject others' suggestions. While they make their expectations clear, they present these as demands. They rarely acknowledge good work. When problems arise, they identify and criticize the culprit. Conflicts are addressed by scapegoating one person as "the problem," which ostracizes her from the rest of the staff. Employees, resentful of this management style, sabotage management's goals or passively resist them. Having learned not to communicate about problems directly, employees backstab supervisors and each other as a way of venting their frustration.

How will each of these nursing home families fare when it comes to the survey process? The very nature of survey preparation demands careful teamwork. A nurturing family facilitates this teamwork by fostering open communication, processing conflict, and providing clear expectations. An inadequate family achieves inconsistent teamwork, because so much depends upon the motivation of individual employees and their teams. A destructive family fosters no teamwork.

As surveyors interact with staff, question residents, and observe staff's communication with one another, they will form an opinion about the kind of "family" you have. If they perceive you as an inadequate or destructive family, they are likely to look for its adverse impact upon resident care.

Possible Solutions

In-services rarely address conflicts among staff and destructive management styles. In-services should educate staff about group processes and communication within an organization. To help you overcome entrenched problems, you could hire an outside consultant. Some outside consultants specialize in team building, which could enhance the working relationships of any group. Finally, nurses could consult with their nursing consultant, and social services staff with their social services consultant. Such an outsider who knows your organization can often provide insight into the problems and make helpful suggestions.

One caution is that, like other systems, nursing home "families" can be resistant to changing. No matter what plan is agreed upon, some staff members may return to their old ways of doing things. That is why any plan for change has to be supported completely by the management team. The team, in turn, must reinforce the changes made by staff and must confront those who show old, destructive behavior.

CONCLUSION

This chapter could have been a very long book in and of itself. We have only discussed surveyors' citations in detail. Readers who wish to learn more about the Resident Assessment Instrument and the process of care planning should consult some of the many books that have been written on these topics.

Part of preparing for survey involves following legal and ethical guidelines in treating residents. These legal and ethical issues are the topic of our next chapter.

REFERENCES

Health Care Financing Administration. (June, 1995). *State operations manual: Provider certification*. Washington, DC: Health Care Finance Administration. (National Technical Information Source No. PB-95-950009.)

Health Care Financing Administration. (October, 1995). *Resident assessment user's manual version 2.0*. Washington, DC: Health Care Finance Administration. (National Technical Information Source No. PB-96-1 09053.)

Institute of Medicine, Committee on Nursing Home Regulation. (1986). *Improving the quality of care in nursing homes*. Wahington, DC: National Acedemy Press.

Chapter 10

Legal and Ethical Issues

Given the prevalence of dementia among LTC residents, staff face many legal and ethical issues. These issues arise at a time when the resident is suffering physically and mentally, and when his relatives are likewise distressed. Consequently, both the resident and family often find it difficult to think clearly about their medical and end-of-life choices. At this point, well-informed staff members can provide invaluable information and feedback. Clear communication with residents and families can help both parties to arrive at satisfactory decisions.

The purpose of this chapter is to help you to become better informed about four legal and ethical issues in LTC: advance directives, competence to make decisions, right-to-die issues, and AMA discharges.

ADVANCE DIRECTIVES

The Patient Self-Determination Act (PSDA) of 1990 was implemented in 1991. This law requires that LTC facilities provide all residents with written information about (1) their rights under state law "to make decisions concerning their medical care, including the right to execute an advance directive," and (2) the facility's procedures for enacting those rights (Dellasega et al., 1996, p. 147). Many facilities fulfill the first requirement by giving patients and families a brochure about medical decision making at the time of admission. PSDA also requires that facilities document in the chart whether a resident has an advance directive, and that they educate staff and members of the community about advance directives.

The term, "advance directives" is an umbrella term for a number of management arrangements made by an elderly person before she becomes incapable of making her own decisions (Grossberg and Zimny, 1996). Included under this umbrella are instruments such as wills, power of attorney, joint ownership, and trusts (Grossberg and Zimny, 1996). In a *living will,* a person makes his wishes known about the use of life-prolonging medical procedures to be implemented if he cannot make or communicate a decision about these. Such procedures include CPR, IV therapy, feeding tubes, respirators and dialysis. Alternatively, a person can execute a *Durable Power of Attorney for Health Care*, in which he names another person, often called an "agent," to make decisions for him. Power of attorney may also be used for other purposes, such as delegating responsibility for handling one's financial affairs. In *joint ownership*, the elderly person directs that the name of another person be placed on financial accounts, with each person's having "full control over the investment and full rights of ownership" (Grossberg and Zimny, 1996, p. 1043).

When residents are admitted who are not capable of informed consent and who have no Durable Power of Attorney for Health Care, it presents a challenging problem for staff, the physician, and family. In this case, the physician and family often agree upon a "preferred intensity of care," which is based upon their knowledge of the resident's past values and preferences. This preferred intensity of care must be described in writing and signed by both the responsible family member and the physician. In cases where the family does not want to complete this form, they often agree upon a do not resuscitate (DNR) order.

Case Illustration

Mr. Smith, who is in a coma, has a Durable Power of Attorney for Health Care indicating that he wants his "life to be prolonged to the greatest extent possible without regard to condition, chances for recovery, or cost." The doctor informs his proxy that Mr. Smith's condition is terminal and death is imminent. Can the agent consent to a DNR order? Must the agent request life-support measures?

The agent cannot request a DNR order. The agent must respect the life-support wishes expressed in the Durable Power of Attorney.

Case Illustration

Mr. Jones, a 95-year-old, long-time resident, has no living family members. Last week he suffered a stroke and then began to refuse food and water. His chart indicates "no code" but there is nothing in his record to indicate his preference for receiving artificial nutrition and hydration. Staff believe that he would not want to be fed with an NG tube, but are not sure whether to withhold that or not.

In this case, his having a "no code" order is irrelevant to the issue of whether he should receive tube feeding. Staff should assess his level of cognitive functioning to determine his decisional ability. If he is capable, then his refusal must be respected. If he is not, the interdisciplinary team should discuss what is known of Mr. Jones and his previous values and preferences. In making a recommendation to the physician, they should take into account his current refusal of food and water.

CAPACITY FOR MAKING MEDICAL AND FINANCIAL DECISIONS

All of the advance directives discussed above must be made while someone is still mentally competent. In defining competence, Miles and Maletta (1996) emphasize the distinction between *decisional ability* and *competence. Competence* is a legal determination made by a court as to whether someone is capable of managing his own affairs. If the person is found incompetent, the court usually assigns someone to manage affairs for him, such as a guardian or conservator. By contrast, *decisional ability* is determined informally by a clinician who assesses a person's ability to make decisions, especially medical and financial ones. While the two terms are often "used interchangeably, the difference emphasizes that limited authority of a clinician over patients who have not yet been declared incompetent and the definitive authority of a designated guardian for a person who has been found incompetent" (Miles and Maletta, 1996, p. 1053). In LTC, decisional ability is the area in which staff's evaluations have an impact. While the attending physician must make the final determination, staff can pool their information at interdisciplinary team meetings and care planning meetings, and can then make a recommendation to the doctor.

In order to be declared decisionally impaired, a patient must have problems that render her unable to "make or communicate responsible decisions" (Grossberg and Zimny, 1996, p. 1053). A diagnostic label alone does not suffice. Specifically, the patient must unable to "(1) receive and communicate information after attempts to reverse or overcome sensory or speech disorders have failed, (2) appreciate the personal implications of risks and benefits, and (3) provide a cogent explanation of how he or she weighs them or relates them to personal goals" (Miles and Maletta, 1996, p. 1053). In addition, staff should be able to demonstrate that she has become more functionally impaired over time, and that she is likely to be substantially harmed because of her inability to manage her affairs (Grossberg and Zimny, 1996). The underlying medical problems that may lead to decisional inability include mental disorders, medical disorders, disability, advanced age, chronic substance abuse, or other disorders (Grossberg and Zimny, 1996).

Decisional ability can vary over time and vary in scope (Miles and Maletta, 1996). The passage of time may show that a person's decisional impairment is "transient and reversible," especially when the cause is a temporary medical condition such as delirium or stress that overwhelms the person (Miles and Maletta, 1996, p. 1054). Concerning the scope of decisional ability, it may be limited to one area of decision making (Miles and Maletta, 1996). For example, a person who cannot evaluate a treatment may be able to decide who should serve as proxy, and one who can make his own medical decisions may still need a financial manager (Miles and Maletta, 1996).

How should staff decide if someone is decisionally capable, and in what areas? Staff must first get an assessment of the person's level of cognitive functioning. To obtain this, staff could refer the resident to their mental health consultant for an opinion. Alternatively, staff could give the Mini-Mental State Exam (MMSE) to get an initial reading. Salthouse (1996) emphasizes that areas measured by the MMSE, such as orientation, attention, and short-term memory, are essential components of one's ability to make rational, informed decisions. Salthouse (1996) suggests that individuals scoring 23 or below "would probably be incapable of making rational decisions" and those scoring 18 or below "would almost certainly not be able" to do so (p. 36). However, he cautions that a score of 24 or more should not be taken as proof that the person is capable. Rather, it should be viewed as a "necessary, rather than sufficient, condition" for rational decision making (Salthouse, 1996, p. 36).

Once staff and the physician decide that someone is decisionally incapable, a "surrogate manager" can be assigned to make decisions on the resident's behalf (Grossberg and Zimny, 1996). A "variety of surrogate management arrangements can be established," and the state laws affecting these vary from state to state (Grossberg and Zimny, 1996, p. 1040). In the instance of nursing home residents, a family member usually becomes the surrogate manager.

Case Illustration

Ms. Carr executed a valid Durable Power of Attorney for Health Care which named her friend, Sam, as proxy. Later, Ms. Carr suffered a severe head injury. Her physician determined that she was not capable of making her own health care decisions. Sam consented to neurosurgery for her, but she refused treatment and became angry with Sam, saying that she no longer wanted him to make decisions for her. Who decides whether to have the surgery?

This is an example of a gray area in bioethics. Usually, in cases like this, staff follow the patient's wishes until a court decides that she is incompetent. To resolve the issue of competence and decision making, Sam could petition the court for a conservatorship of person with medical provisions. If Ms. Carr is deemed competent, she can revoke him as proxy. If deemed incompetent, she cannot revoke him. If he is granted full authority to provide medical consent, he can overrule her objection to surgery. In cases like this, staff should inform the ombudsman and ask for a review by the facility's bioethics committee.

RIGHT-TO-DIE ISSUES

About 1.5 million deaths occur in the United States each year because life-sustaining treatment is withheld or withdrawn (Miles and Miletta, 1996). In order for staff to withhold or withdraw such treatment legally, the following standards must be met: (a) all lifesustaining treatments, including food and fluids, are elective; (b) the patient or proxy must give consent; and (c) the patient need not have an irreversible illness in order to refuse treatment (Miles and Maletta, 1996). In enforcing these standards, "states vary as to the degree of proof that is required for evidence of an incompetent person's preference to forego treatment" (Miles and Maletta, 1996, p. 1055).

One concern is that residents who choose to forego lifesustaining treatment may be depressed and thus have a perspective on life that is too pessimistic. Residents with severe medical problems are often appropriately sad and subclinically depressed. In these cases, the resident's mood is probably not clouding her judgement to a significant degree (Miles and Maletta, 1996). However, when a resident scores 11 or more on the Geriatric Depression Scale and reports a clinical level of depressive symptoms, she may be viewing the world through very dark glasses. In this case, staff can attempt to treat her depression, with the hope that improved mood will create a more balanced perspective. If her depression does not improve with intervention, staff have to weigh all the factors involved, such as the patient's prior values, cognitive ability, advance directives, and/or the wishes of family members.

One of the most difficult decisions for staff to make is whether a patient's medical condition is potentially reversible or not. When the patient is decisionally incapable and reversibility is unclear, Chicin (1995) suggests that staff provide a "time-limited trial of treatment" to see if his condition improves (p. 41). If not, "the staff has the comfort of realizing they have tried every possible intervention" (Chicin, 1995, p. 41). Chicin (1995) does acknowledge that "it is often far more difficult, on an emotional level, for health care providers to withdraw a treatment than it is to withhold the same treatment" (p. 42). However, "most ethicists agree that there is no moral or ethical difference" (Chicin, 1995, p. 42).

Finally, throughout the process, it is important for staff to acknowledge their own feelings for the patient. Staff members often develop feelings of affection for their patients, becoming "surrogate family to the residents for whom they care" (Chicin, 1995, p. 41). Consequently, many staff "who accept a patient's right" to die "on an intellectual level have great difficulty on an emotional level," especially when the patient is decisionally incapable (Chicin, 1995, p. 41). Because of this difficulty, staff need to be supported as they withdraw or withhold treatment, and they may need to be reminded of the resident's right to make such a decision (Chicin, 1995).

Case Study

Ms. C, an 89-year-old resident, was referred for psychological assessment of her depression and cognitive ability to make her own medical decisions. The presenting problem was that she was giving contradictory messages to her physician about her will to live and her willingness to have a G-tube.

Specifically, she had suffered a stroke about six weeks prior to the evaluation, which made her unable to swallow and made it difficult for her to talk. While receiving therapy for her dysphagia, she was fed by an IV line, which she had told staff that she wanted. However, her family members protested, saying that she had told them that she wanted it taken out so that she could die. The attending physician responded that she could not take action without hearing a clear message from her. Several days later, she told her physician that she did not want any form of artificial nutrition, either intravenous or via a G-tube. However, later that day, she said that she wanted the IV line to stay in until the next day. The next day she said that she wanted to continue her therapy and to have a G-tube inserted until she could resume eating.

At this point, the psychological assessment was requested. She admitted sadness about having to "lie here day after day," about not making progress in her therapy, and about "praying for a total cure and nothing happens." However, she denied crying, insomnia, or wishing she were dead. She did not test as clinically depressed on the Geriatric Depression Scale. Cognitive screening suggested mild dementia. Concerning her swallowing, she said that she wanted the G-tube because her doctor recommended it. However, she admitted that it was difficult for her to accept the procedure.

The psychologist concluded that she displayed intermittent, mild depression and mild cognitive impairment. The psychologist noted that her contradictory messages were probably caused by her fluctuating mood and mildly impaired memory. She seemed more likely to have requested withdrawal of nutrition when depressed, and both her mood and memory problems may have prevented her from recalling what she had previously said. The psychologist recommended that staff continue to check regularly with her about her will to live and her desire for the G-tube. He explained to her relatives that staff needed to hear consistent messages from her about what she wanted. Psychotherapy was not recommended because of her difficulty talking.

Over the next two weeks, she told staff consistently that she wanted a G-tube and thus she received one. Her mood improved, especially because she made progress in her therapy. However, during the ensuing two weeks, her progress in therapy slowed and she became more discouraged. She continued to need the G-tube for feeding, and she said that she wished she did not need it. Her mood continued to fluctuate from day to day. Over the next week, she decided that she no longer wanted to live, and gave staff consistent messages about no longer wanting the G-tube. Her physician ordered the G-tube removed, and she signed over her benefits to the hospice program.

THE BIOETHICS COMMITTEE

In order to address cases like those above, a bioethics committee can be formed. The purposes of this committee are to ensure that all sides of an issue are explored before a decision is made, to ensure that the rights and best interests of residents are honored, and to provide the facility with documentation that it has formally reviewed all difficult cases. The committee can be composed of the following members: Administrator, Director of Nursing, Medical Director or attending physician, Social Services Director, Ombudsman, and in some cases, a relative, and the Mental Health Consultant.

The committee meets only when a specific legal or ethical issue arises for a given resident. Examples of such issues are provided above. Other issues that might cause the committee to meet include: disagreement among family members about the type of treatment a resident should receive, a case in which the resident is related to her physician or to staff members at the facility, a case in which the resident is supervised by a public guardian, and issues of confidentiality. As committee members discuss each case, their goal is to make judgements that are consistent with the resident's explicit wishes and implicit values, to the extent they are known. The committee should keep minutes for each meeting, and its recommendations should be documented in the patient's medical record.

AMA DISCHARGES

Sooner or later in your work in LTC, you will have a resident who wants to check himself out "against medical advice" (AMA). Sometimes a competent resident who is alcoholic checks himself out AMA in order to resume drinking. In other cases, a nonconserved resident who has no family members to sign for him decides to check himself out AMA.

Regardless of the reason, staff should first explain to the resident why they think it is in her best interest to stay at the home. If that fails, staff should (1) have the resident sign an AMA discharge form, and (2) notify the Ombudsman. In many cases staff should also notify Adult Protective Services (APS). If the resident is homeless upon discharge, staff should notify the county employee who coordinates services for the homeless or who serves as a "street" mental health worker. If the resident is returning to her home, they can refer her to a home health care organization. The following case illustrates some of the issues and actions necessary with an AMA discharge.

Case Study

Ms. H, an 80-year-old female resident with Alzheimer's dementia and hypothyroidism was referred for psychological assessment after having almost signed herself out AMA two days before. She had stopped short of signing herself out because she was not able to understand the AMA discharge form that she was to sign. She had no surviving relatives, was not conserved, and had no agent designated by a Durable Power of Attorney. Thus, she was the only one who could make medical decisions for herself. The referral question was whether she was cognitively capable of understanding the form and whether the assessing professional could engage her in a reasonable discussion of the pros and cons of returning home, so that she might decide to stay at the nursing home voluntarily.

She had been admitted to the nursing home four months previously because she had fallen in her apartment while carrying groceries, and had lain there for over two days until someone finally heard her cries for help. She was then admitted to the hospital, where she was treated for urinary tract infection and dehydration. While at the hospital, she said that she wanted to return home, which staff thought would place her at severe risk. Thus, the hospital staff contacted Adult Protective Services, who assigned a worker to the case. This APS worker continued to follow her when she was transferred to the nursing home. She had continued to pay rent at this apartment during the time she lived at the nursing home; thus, it was still available to her.

While at the home, she frequently became lost as she wandered the halls, and at times, she had attempted to leave. Nursing notes indicated that she needed assistance with her ADLs, was at risk for falls, experienced back pain, and needed her thyroid problem monitored closely. Despite these problems, she continued to tell staff that she wanted to go home. Thus, the APS worker decided to refer her to the Public Guardian's office for a conservatorship application.

When she was confronted with these medical needs during the interview, she became angry and denied all of them, saying, "That's ridiculous! Who could say that?" She reiterated that she wanted to return to her apartment very badly. Testing with the Geriatric Depression Scale showed a score of 4, indicating no clinical depression, and she denied having depression during the interview. While cognitive screening suggested average functioning in seven areas, it also showed severely impaired orientation, mildly impaired comprehension, moderately impaired recent memory, and moderately impaired construction. Given this impairment and her adamant denial of her medical problems, her insight was considered poor. Overall, the findings were consistent with her diagnosis of Alzheimer's dementia.

The psychologist concluded that she was not capable of understanding the AMA discharge form, or of weighing the pros and cons of returning home. He recommended that staff continue their conservatorship application, and that they consult with the corporation's attorney to explore any options for keeping her at the home. The attorney said that if she chose to leave prior to the completion of the conservatorship application, staff would have to let her sign herself out.

Several days after the evaluation, she did sign herself out AMA and returned to her apartment by taxicab. Upon discharge, the social services assistant gave her a list of community resources, and notified her

APS worker, her apartment manager, the APS staff member on call, the Public Guardian's office, and the ombudsman. The Assistant documented all of this in the chart.

CONCLUSION

These are difficult, often controversial issues that can divide staff as much as they do families, especially when staff feel attached to the resident and believe that they know what is best for him. Hopefully, as you become more acquainted with current legal and ethical thinking in these areas, you can develop a philosophy that you as a staff can live with. That, in turn, will help you to communicate more clearly and consistently with residents and families.

Dealing with these difficult, often emotional issues adds to the strain of working in LTC. Unfortunately, it is only one reason why so many staff feel stressed and burned out while working in this field. Helping staff to reduce this stress and burnout is the topic of our final chapter.

REFERENCES

Chicin, E.R. (1995). Treatment termination in long-term care: Implications for health care providers. In E. Olsen, E.R. Chicin, and L.S. Libow (Eds.), *Controversies in ethics in long-term care* (pp. 29-42). New York: Springer.

Dellasega, C., Smyer, M., Frank, L., and Brown, R. (1996). Commentary: Decision-making capacity in the acutely ill elderly. In M. Smyer, K.W. Schaie, and M.B. Kapp (Eds.), *Older adults' decision-making and the law* (pp. 142-161). New York: Springer.

Grossberg, G.T. and Zimny, G.H. (1996). Medical-legal issues. In J. Sadavoy, L.W. Lazarus, L.F. Jarvik, and G.T. Grossberg (Eds.), *Comprehensive review of geriatric psychiatry II* (3rd edition, pp. 1037-1050). Washington, DC: American Psychiatric Press.

Miles, S.H., and Maletta, G. (1996). Clinical ethics. In Sadavoy, L.W. Lazarus, L.F. Jarvik, and G.T. Grossberg (Eds.), *Comprehensive review of geriatric psychiatry II* (3rd edition, pp. 1051-1064). Washington, DC: American Psychiatric Press.

Patient Self-Determination Act, Omnibus Budget Reconciliation Act of 1990, Public Law Number 101-508, Section 4206, 4751.

Salthouse, T.A. (1996). Commentary: A cognitive psychologist's perspective on the assessment of cognitive competency. In M. Smyer, K.W. Schaie, and M.B. Kapp (Eds.), *Older adults' decision-making and the law* (pp. 29-39). New York: Springer.

Chapter 11

Preventing Burnout:
Taking Care of Your Own
Psychosocial Needs

We now come to perhaps the most important topic in this book: your own psychosocial needs. We believe that you cannot serve others effectively unless you are taking care of yourself. If you are demoralized, dead-tired, preoccupied, and irritable, you will be far less effective with residents and other staff. All that toxic emotion may prevent you from applying your knowledge and skills and working with other members of the team.

Burnout affects everyone in the nursing home, because it contributes to staff turnover, absenteeism, and low morale (Maslach and Jackson, 1986). As staff constantly leave their jobs, call in sick, or complain, everyone's motivation for work suffers. In addition, residents suffer when they lose trusted caregivers to turnover or receive substandard treatment from staff who no longer care.

In this chapter, we ask that you reflect on the question, "How well am I taking care of myself and how can I do it better?" To help you do so, we describe symptoms of burnout, common causes of burnout in LTC, and proactive steps that you can take to protect and nurture your own emotional health.

SYMPTOMS OF BURNOUT

In their book, *When Helping Starts to Hurt*, Grosch and Olsen describe burnout as an "erosion of the spirit" in which staff lose "faith in the very enterprise of helping" (1994, p. 4). Staff are most likely to burn out when they take on a helping role with "high ideals and commitment," only to have these melt into "disillusion or even cynicism" (p. 4). This disillusionment "manifests itself in a variety of ways, ranging from a sense of personal deadness, dragging through the days, watching the clock, dreading seeing another client, to a complete breakdown and inability to go on" (pp. ix-x). The authors liken this inability to go on to a marathon runner's "hitting the wall," which is the point in the race at which he feels that he cannot take another step.

More specifically, there are three primary dimensions to burnout: *emotional exhaustion, depersonalization,* and a *reduced sense of personal accomplishment* (Maslach and Jackson,1986). Of these three dimensions, depersonalization needs definition. "Depersonalization" entails "negative, cynical attitudes" toward residents and a "callous or even dehumanized perception" of them (Maslach and Jackson, 1986, p. 1). Staff may depersonalize residents by treating them as impersonal objects or by no longer caring about their quality of care (Maslach and Jackson, 1986). The burden of paperwork in LTC often contributes to this impersonal treatment of residents, as they often become just one more stop on the papermill assembly line.

Burnout is not the same as depression. Depression can co-exist with burnout, but it does not have to. There is some evidence that when depression does accompany burnout, it usually arrives after the burnout has festered for a while (McKnight and Glass, 1995). In other words, it is more likely that a burned-out person will become depressed than that a depressed person will become burned out. This points out yet another reason why we believe that this chapter is so important: not only do we want to help you to prevent burnout, but in doing so, we hope to prevent the depression that may follow.

CAUSES OF BURNOUT

One source of burnout is quite obvious: job stress. As shown in Table 11.1, there are many sources of stress for those who work in LTC.

Keep in mind, however, that burnout can be also be caused by stressors originating at home. Some studies have shown that burnout is more related to marital problems that to work stress (Pines and

TABLE 11.1. Sources of Stress in Long-Term Care

General Sources	Specific Sources
Environment	Noise, odors, poor lighting, poor ventilation, cramped offices, lack of privacy for staff.
Few tangible rewards	Low or modest pay, bonuses are rare, few promotional opportunities.
Workload	Too many demands, too little time for residents, skipping breaks and lunch, having little control over job responsibilities.
Need for emotional self-control	Need to maintain tact with residents and family members despite inner feelings.
Residents	Present very difficult problems, rarely express appreciation, can be irritating, force us to face old age and death.
Family members	Can be overly demanding and critical, may abandon or neglect their relative.
Other staff members	Conflicts among staff, poor support or recognition from management.

Aronson, 1988 as cited in Grosch and Olsen, 1994). If you arrive at work distressed by last night's argument, chances are better that you will find the day's demands overwhelming and irritating. Some people with stressful marriages try to escape by immersing themselves in long hours of work (Grosch and Olsen, 1994). Others seek the affirmation at work that they do not get at home, which often leads to disappointment.

Trying to meet the demands of both family and work can also lead to burnout. A recent study of nurses in an LTC facility showed that those who felt torn between their family and work responsibilities were most likely to burn out (Ray and Miller, 1994). Specifically, those nurses who were mothers, or who were unmarried but living with someone, were more likely to display burnout. In discussing their findings, the authors point out that women working in human services are often "nurturing, empathic, and sensitive to others.

When they have to balance home and work, they often find they give to everyone but themselves" (Ray and Miller, 1994, p. 362).

Of course, one motive for helping others may be the "deep desire to be liked and admired which can easily drive us to overwork" (Grosch and Olsen, 1994, p. 117). Grosch and Olsen point out that many of us choose helping roles "not out of a genuine concern for others, but rather out of a need to be appreciated by them" (1994, p. 117). These strong desires for approval, appreciation, and admiration can lead us to disappointment in our work in LTC. We may have entered the field expecting that the residents or family members would acknowledge our efforts on their behalf. Instead, they often do not understand our workload demands or appreciate our extra efforts. Consequently, we feel empty and frustrated.

Finally, lack of support from upper management places staff at greater risk for burnout. The study discussed above showed that the LTC nurses were much more likely to burn out if they believed that their supervisors or administrator gave them little support, respect, or appreciation (Ray and Miller, 1994).

TREATING AND PREVENTING BURNOUT

Before we discuss solutions to burnout, we must address a barrier to getting help: shame. Grosch and Olsen (1994) emphasize that many helping professionals have a "fantasy of omnipotent helpfulness and resist every effort to create doubt about its validity" (p. 147). When burnout reveals the cracks in this fantasy, they are ashamed "because they feel that they have failed in the arena where they are most proud" (p. 144). They are embarrassed to realize that their "selfless devotion" was really a way of gaining others' admirations and appreciation (Grosch and Olsen, 1994). Acknowledging and getting past this shame and embarrassment opens the door to healing.

Once staff acknowledge that they are beginning to burn out, a number of interventions are possible, such as changing jobs within the organization, joining a support group, or starting personal psychotherapy (Grosch and Olsen, 1994). Psychotherapy can provide a forum for exploring your motives for helping others, for identifying what your most important needs are, and for coming up with possible solutions. You may conclude that you are expecting too much from yourself, or that you are expecting to get more appreciation for what you do than is realistic. On the other hand, you may decide that working in LTC does not fit your personal interests and needs.

Sometimes taking more time off from work is helpful. However, if the real problem is frustration with the organization, having too many responsibilities, or not feeling appreciated, then time off may not help. In these cases, you may dread returning to work, and every vacation may seem too short. On the other hand, getting away can sometimes provide you with enough emotional distance that you think of new ideas and solutions.

Changing Organizational Causes of Burnout

A key source of burnout is the organization, including its demands on staff and the quality of its management. To address organizational concerns, staff can start by sharing their feelings with co-workers "to find out the extent of burnout that others in the organization are experiencing" (Grosch and Olsen, 1994, p. 137). In doing so, they can pinpoint problems within the organization that should be solved. For example, staff members "can bargain to modify or reduce caseloads, urge or propose modifications in burdensome chart procedures, identify and speak to or complain about unhelpful supervisors . . . " (Grosch and Olsen, 1994, p. 137).

Workload Changes

Proposing modifications that reduce your workload requires the utmost in forethought, tact, and negotiating skill. For this reason, you should begin by discussing the most burdensome areas with other employees. As a group, you can think of ways to make changes that will lighten the load but preserve the quality and timeliness of care. You can then present your ideas to the appropriate supervisor. Many staff find it helpful to first discuss their issues with the social services or nurse consultant. Sometimes this consultant can raise the issues with the administration, or can facilitate negotiation between staff and management.

If you are a parent who feels torn between the demands of work and family, you will have to look carefully at the causes of the problem. If you decide that the nature of your work in LTC contributes to the home/work tension, then you may wish to approach management about ways to ease the burden. For example, you could ask for an alternative work schedule or flexible work hours.

Many staff are reluctant to propose changes, because they fear that supervisors will perceive them as insubordinate. Such is not likely if you propose changes that incorporate your supervisor's goals and priorities–if you present the changes as a proposal and not as a demand, and if you are willing to negotiate. In addition, presenting the proposal as a group or with the help of your consultant makes it less likely that one of you will be seen as insubordinate.

Improving Management and Teamwork

As we noted, unsupportive and unappreciative managers are a key reason for staff's burning out. Often poor management leads to the "inadequate" or "destructive" nursing home "family" described in Chapter 9. Within teams, constant conflict among staff members is demoralizing and emotionally wearing. It can lead to the obvious question: "How can we take care of residents' needs when we cannot get along with each other?"

In Chapter 9, we made a number of recommendations for addressing the problems of poor management and teamwork. These included in-service training in work group dynamics and the use of outside management consultants.

When it comes to addressing concerns about specific managers or team members, talking with them directly is an important first step. If that fails, you can discuss the problem with that person's supervisor. Once again, speaking up as a group gives you more power than doing it alone.

Of course, many staff members do not trust their managers or team members enough to ask for changes. They believe that they will receive an apathetic or hostile response. However, we believe that wherever possible, staff should make a clear attempt to negotiate change before assuming that such is not possible. Even the most difficult person can sometimes be receptive. If these attempts fail, then asking for an outside consultant is appropriate. If that does not work, you may have to pursue a job in a more supportive work section or facility.

Developing Your Skills and Expertise

Work in LTC can become boring and routine if your skills do not grow. For this reason, Szwabo and Stein (1993) underscore the importance of "staff development and educational programs to continually update and enhance knowledge of caregivers" (p. 251). When you learn new skills and approaches, you can become more energized at work because you have "new toys" to try out. New skills also provide you with greater hope for better future jobs or promotions.

Similarly, developing a special area of expertise or interest can make work more interesting. In his study of professionals who recovered from burnout, Cherniss (1995) found that those who recovered most had developed a "unique project, program, or specialty" that was "simulating and meaningful" (p. 126). In LTC nursing, there are a number of areas that might serve as specialties, such as Total Quality Improvement, hospice, legal and ethical issues, comfort care, and psychiatric nursing. Such specialty areas can help staff to attain "high levels of autonomy, challenge, responsibility, and meaning" (Cherniss, 1995, p. 127).

A Spiritual Perspective

Grosch and Olsen (1994) underscore the importance of "spiritual refreshment" and "nurturing one's spiritual self." Obviously, sustaining one's self spiritually means vastly different things to different people. Regardless of the spiritual path, the main reason why spiritual nurturance is so important is that it can give us a renewed sense of meaning and purpose. A spiritual perspective reminds us that we are part of a larger, more meaningful picture, even when we feel discouraged or powerless as individuals. Armed with a "transcendent" perspective that takes us beyond our "egoistic" motives, we can endure stressful work much more easily (Cherniss, 1995, p. 185).

There are two reasons why a spiritual perspective is particularly important for those working in LTC. First, a spiritual perspective often provides a moral reason for caring, and it is our ability to care that most often suffers when we are burning out. This perspective may enable us to care even when we are not getting external appreciation for our efforts. Here, we are the ones who can praise ourselves for living consistently with our own moral and spiritual standards. Second, we are confronted daily with sickness and death, which forces us to face our own vulnerability. A spiritual perspective can help us to face this vulnerability without feeling as threatened.

Time Management Techniques

Sometimes staff burnout because they have a mountain of things to do and work extra, unpaid hours to keep up. In this case, time management techniques become extremely important. We offer four ideas for better managing your time.

Set Limits and Boundaries

Nursing homes can be as chaotic as they are demanding. No staff member can be available to everyone all of the time. At care-planning conferences, put a clock on the table and reach an agreement with co-workers about how much time will be allowed for reviewing each care plan. If family members or residents have concerns that cannot be addressed in the time allotted, schedule appointments for another time. Having voice mail or an answering machine is another way to set boundaries. Such can help prevent your being paged constantly and can allow you to screen calls and return them at convenient times.

Delegate Responsibility

Sometimes staff do work that others could or should be doing. Look critically at what you do each week and ask yourself whether any of it could be assigned to another person. Volunteers or family members may be able to help a resident with shopping, taking an inventory of her possessions, or keeping medical appointments. If other staff members in your department or on your shift do not do their share of the work, raise the issue with them or with management. If you are doing work that another agency should be doing, take steps to shift the responsibility to that agency. For example, a social services designee was doing lots of discharge planning on behalf of an assisted living center, to which her LTC residents were often referred. This proved to be a burdensome addition to her workload, and in fact, was benefiting the assisted living center more than her own home. Her social services consultant recommended that she have staff from the assisted living do the discharge planning, which relieved her of most of the extra work.

Get Organized

A messy and cluttered office makes it difficult to keep your paperwork organized, and gives others the impression that you are not organized. Make a daily "to do" list and prioritize it by tackling the tough assignments first. To ensure adequate time for charting, some staff come in early one or two days a week when things are quiet. Finally, make a weekly calendar with blocked-out times for meetings, office time, and lunch. Some staff put this calendar on their door so that residents, staff, and families know where they are and when they are available to see them.

Keep a Log

Set up a binder with alphabetized dividers and place a face sheet and a blank log sheet in it for each resident. The face sheet gives you instant demographic data for each resident. Each log sheet should have space at the top for your care plans, so that you are reminded of the specific interventions for that resident. When you do weekly rounds, use the log to record what is needed for the resident and what interventions were made. At the end of each week, write down interventions from the log book so that they can be later transferred to your quarterly report. While this may consume more time in the short run, it will save time during the writing of quarterly reports, and it may improve their accuracy.

Use a Computer

With a computer and a word processing program, you can place your key documents for each resident on a computer file. These may include care plans, intake summaries, assessments, and quarterly reports. Once the initial documents are completed, revising them for subsequent reports often requires less time than completing a new form.

CONCLUSION

Preventing burnout is easier than treating it after it has festered for a while. Working in LTC places you at high risk for burnout, which means that you must take aggressive steps to take care of yourself. Often the most difficult step is to acknowledge your own needs and vulnerability. After that, you can address your own psychosocial needs without shame or hesitation. Taking practical steps to care for your own needs, such as those described above, is essential. Ultimately, however, it may be your ability to find a transcendent meaning in your work that determines whether you flourish or languish in LTC.

REFERENCES

Cherniss, C. (1995). *Beyond burnout: Helping teachers, nurses, therapists, and lawyers recover from stress and disillusionment.* New York: Routledge.

Grosch, W.N. and Olsen, D.C. (1994). *When helping starts to hurt: A new look at burnout among psychotherapists.* New York: W.W. Norton and Company.

Maslach, C. and Jackson, S.E. (1986). *Maslach burnout inventory,* Second Edition (Manual). Palo Alto, CA: Consulting Psychologists Press.

McKnight, J.D. and Glass, D.C. (1995). Perceptions of control, burnout, and depressive symptomatology. *Journal of Consulting and Clinical Psychology,* 63, 490-494.

Pines, A. and Aronson, E. (1988). *Career burnout: Causes and cures* (2nd edition). New York: Free Press.

Ray, E.B. and Miller, K.I. (1994). Social support, home/work stress, and burnout: Who can help? *Journal of Applied Behavioral Science,* 30, 357-373.

Szwabo, P.A. and Stein, A.L. (1993). Professional care-giver stress in long-term care. In P.A. Szwabo and G.T. Grossberg (Eds.), *Problem behaviors in long-term care: Diagnosis and treatment* (pp. 242-253). New York: Springer.

Appendixes

APPENDIX A

Care Plan Resources

Beard, D.J. and Greenwald, S.C. *The social work care plan training manual: A comprehensive guide to meeting the OBRA requirements.* Bossier City, LA: Professional Printing.

Davis, E.J. and Greenwald, S.C. (1991). *The care plan answer book for activities, psychosocial, and social services programs.* Stokie, IL: SCG Consulting/Publishing.

Giacopuzzi, J. *Patient care plan problems for social services.* (Available from Psychosocial Consultants, 13506 Hike Lane, San Diego, CA 92129.)

Hughes, M. and Espinosa, M. (1993). *Revised social service care plans for nursing homes.* Bossier City, LA: Professional Printing.

March, C.S. (1992). *The complete care plan manual for long-term care.* (Available from American Hospital Publishing, Inc., 800-AHA-2626)

APPENDIX B

Responsibilities of the Social Services Department*

A. Regardless of size, all facilities are required to provide for the medically related social service needs of each resident. This requirement specifies that facilities aggressively identify the need for medically related social services, and pursue the provision of these services...

B. "Medically related social services" means services provided by the facility's staff to assist residents in maintaining or improving their ability to manage their everyday physical, mental, and psychological needs. These services might include, for example:

1. Making arrangements for obtaining needed adaptive equipment, clothing, and personal items;

2. Maintaining contact with family (with resident's permission) to report on changes in health, current goals, discharge planning, and encouragement to participate in care planning;

3. Assisting staff to inform residents and those they designate about the resident's health status and health care choices and their ramifications;

4. Making referrals and obtaining services from outside entities (e.g., talking books, absentee ballots, community wheelchair transportation);

5. Assisting residents with financial and legal matters (e.g., applying for pensions, referrals to lawyers, referrals to funeral homes for preplanning arrangements);

6. Discharge planning services (e.g., helping to place a resident on a waiting list for community congregate living, arranging intake for home care services for residents returning home, assisting with transfer arrangements to other facilities);

7. Providing or arranging provision of needed counseling services;

---

*From "Guidance to Surveyors," Section 483.15 (g) (1).

8. Through the assessment and care planning process, identifying and seeking ways to support resident's individual needs and preferences, customary routines, concerns and choices;

9. Building relationships between residents and staff and teaching staff how to understand and support residents' individual needs;

10. Promoting actions by staff that maintain or enhance each resident's dignity in full recognition of each resident's individuality;

11. Assisting residents to determine how they would like to make decisions about their health care, and whether or not they would like anyone else to be involved in those decisions;

12. Finding options that most meet the physical and emotional needs of each resident;

13. Providing alternatives to drug therapy or restraints by understanding and communicating to staff why residents act as they do, what they are attempting to communicate, and what needs the staff must meet;

14. Meeting the needs of the residents who are grieving; and

15. Finding options which most meet their physical and emotional needs.

C. Factors with a potentially negative effect on physical, mental, and psychosocial well-being include an unmet need for:

1. Dental/denture care;
2. Podiatric care;
3. Eye care;
4. Hearing services;
5. Equipment for mobility or assistive eating devices; and
6. Need for home-like environment, control, dignity, privacy.

D. Where needed services are not covered by the Medicaid State Plan, nursing facilities are still required to attempt to obtain these services. For example, if a resident requires transportation services that are not covered under a State Medicaid Plan, the facility is required to provide these services. This could be achieved, for example, through obtaining volunteer assistance.

E. Types of conditions to which the facility should respond with social services include:

1. Lack of an effective family/social support system;

2. Behavioral symptoms;

3. If a resident with dementia strikes out at another resident, the facility should evaluate the resident's behavior...

4. Presence of a chronic disabling medical or psychological condition (e.g., multiple sclerosis, chronic obstructive pulmonary disease, Alzheimer's disease, schizophrenia);

5. Depression;

6. Chronic or acute pain;

7. Difficulty with personal interaction and socialization skills;

8. Presence of legal or financial problems;

9. Abuse of alcohol or other drugs;

10. Inability to cope with loss of function;

11. Need for emotional support;

12. Changes in family relationships, living arrangements and/or resident's condition or functioning; and

13. A physical or chemical restraint.

F. Probes: Section 483.15 (g) (1) For residents selected for a comprehensive or focused review as appropriate:

1. How do facility staff implement social services interventions to assist the resident in meeting treatment goals?

2. How do staff responsible for social work monitor the resident's programs in improving physical, mental, and psychosocial functioning? Has goal attainment been evaluated and care plan changed accordingly?

3. How does the care plan link goals to psychosocial functioning/well-being?

4. Have the staff responsible for social work established and maintained relationships with the resident's family or legal representative?

5. [NFs] What attempts do the facility make to access services for Medicaid recipients when those services are not covered by a Medicaid State Plan?

G. Look for evidence that social services interventions successfully address residents' needs and link social supports, physical care, and physical environment with residents' needs and individuality.

H. For sampled residents, review MDS, section H.

Note: Excerpted from HCFA June, 1995.

APPENDIX C

Quality of Life Assessment:
Individual and Group Interview Questions
for HCFA Surveyors

Topic	Types of Questions
1. Room and Building	•How are the light and temperature in your room? •How is the air circultion? •What do you think of the noise level here? •Do you ever see insects or rodents here? •Is the facility clean and free of bad smells? •If you ever changed rooms, what was the reason and did you have a choice about changing rooms? •Do staff here try to make it homelike here?
2. Privacy	•Does the staff respect your privacy? •Can you meet privately with visitors? •Do you have privacy when on the telephone?
3. Food	•How does your food taste? •How is the temperature of your food? •If you ever refused to eat something served to you, and did staff offer you something else?
4. Activities	•How do you find out about activities that are going on? •Do you participate in and enjoy activities? •Are there enough help and supplies available so that everyone who wants to can participate? •Do you have a say in the activities offered?

Topic	Types of Questions
5. Staff	•Do staff treat you with respect? •Do they make the effort to listen to and resolve your problems? •Has any resident or staff member ever physically harmed you? •Has a staff member ever yelled or sworn at you? •Are there enough staff here to care for everyone?
6. ADLs	•Do you get help when you need it? •Do staff encourage you to do as much as you can for yourself?
7. Decisions	•Are you involved in making decisions about your nursing care and medical treatment? •If you want to change your care or daily schedule, how do you let staff know? •Do staff members respond to your requests?
8. Medical Services	•Are you satisfied with your physician's care? •Do you have privacy when examined by your physician? •Do staff help you to make appointments and to obtain transportation?
9. Rules	•Tell me about the rules in this facility. •Do you have input into the rules?
10. Personal Belongings	•How are your personal belongings treated here? •Have any of your belongings ever been missing?

Topic	Types of Questions
11. Rights	•How do you find out about your rights?
	•Are you invited to meetings in which staff plan your medical care, treatment, and activities?
	•Do you know how to contact an advocate like the ombudsman?
	•Do you know that you can look at your medical record?
	•Tell me about the mail delivery system here.
	•Have you voiced a grievance to the facility, and if so, how did staff respond?
12. Dignity	•How do staff members treat residents here?
	•Do staff treat residents with respect and dignity?
13. Costs	•Are you informed about which items are paid by Medicare or Medicaid and which ones you must pay for?
	•Are you aware of any changes in the care residents have received after they went from paying for their care to Medicaid's paying?
14. Council	•Do staff help you with arrangements for council meetings?
	•How does the council communicate its concerns to the staff?
	•How does the administrator respond to the council's concerns?

Source: Adapted from Forms HCFA-806 and HCFA-806A, July, 1995. Most questions are paraphrased.

APPENDIX D

Quality of Life Assessment:
Observation of Noninterviewable Resident
for HCFA Surveyors

Topic	Examples of what is observed
Resident and Environment	Appearance, level of assistance received, privacy during care, use of restraints, staff's response when resident indicates needs.
Daily Life	Concordance between daily activities and resident's interests and functional level. Is the resident given choices, e.g., concerning food and drink, or radio and TV being on?
Interactions	Degree to which staff tailor their interactions to the resident's needs and interests, resident's response to staff's communication, opportunities for socializing, evidence of roommate problems.

Source: Adapted from Form HCFA-806C, July, 1995. Most statements are paraphrased.

APPENDIX E

Quality of Life Assessment: Family Interview Questions for HCFA Surveyors

Topic	**Types of Questions**
Nature and extent of relatiorship between interviewee and resident	How often did you see your relative prior to this placement, and how often now?
Lifestyle and preferences when he/she was more independent.	Are you familiar with your relative's preferences and daily routines when he/she was more independent? For example, what were his/her activities, interests, and eating and sleeping habits?
Resident's lifelong general personality	How did he/she adapt to change prior to the disability?
Changes in preferences and personality after LTC placement	Have any of his/her daily activities or routines changed since moving here?
Observations, positive and negative, about the facility	Topics: meals, activities, visitation policies, quality of nursing care, noise, privacy during care, transfers, security, cleanliness/odors.
Interviewee's participation in the admission process	What, if anything, did they tell you about using Medicare or Medicaid to pay for the stay or for extra services above the Medicaid rate?
Notification of changes in condition	If you are the person to be notified, have you been notified of changes in the resident's condition? Are you involved in care planning?

Source: Adapted from Form HCFA-806C, July, 1995. Most questions are paraphrased.

APPENDIX F

Resident Review Worksheet
for Surveyors

Topic	Examples of Issues Evaluated
Resident's Room	• Adequate privacy, call bells functioning, accessible bathroom, resident with physical limitations can move in his/her room, homelike and comfortable environment, comfortable temperature, good lighting.
Resident Daily Life Review	• Grooming, quality of communication with staff, staff's response to requests and call bells, freedom from unexplained injuries, activities tailored to resident's needs, provision of medically related social services, necessity of restraints (if used).
Drug Therapies	• Rationale, side effects, dose, monitoring. • Evidence of unnecessary medications, including antipsychotic drugs. • What is relationship between drug therapy and clinical condition?
RAI/Care Review Sheet	• For a *comprehensive review*: complete an overall review of the RAI including all ADL functional areas, cognitive status, and MDS categories triggering a RAP. • For a *focused review:* **Phase 1:** Complete a review of those requirements for concerns and care areas specific to the resident. **Phase 2:** Complete a review of requirements appropriate to concern areas.

Topic	Examples of Issues Evaluated
RAI/Care Review Sheet (continued)	• If the RAI is less than nine months old, scan and compare with the previous RAI and most recent quarterly review. If the RAI is nine months or older, compare the current RAI with the most recent quarterly review. Note any differences for the applicable areas being reviewed.
	• Review the RAP summary and care planning. Look for implementation of the care plan. Note specifically the effects of care or lack of care. If the resident declined or failed to improve relative to expectations, determine if this was avoidable or unavoidable.

Source: Adapted from Form HCFA-805, July, 1995. Many statements are paraphrased.

APPENDIX G

General Observations About the Facility

Topic	Examples of Issues Evaluated
Handrails	Do corridors have handrails?
Odors	Is the facility free of objectionable odors and well ventilated?
Cleanliness	How clean is the environment?
Pests	Is the facility pest-free?
Linen	Is linen processed properly to prevent the spread of infection?
Hazards	Is the facility as free of accident hazards as possible?
Call System	Is there a functioning call system in bathing areas and in resident toilets in common areas?
Space	Are the space and furnishings in dining and activity areas sufficient to accommodate all activities?
Furnishings	Are dining and activity rooms adequately furnished?
Drug storage	Are drugs and biologicals stored properly?
Equipment	Is the resident equipment in common areas sanitary, orderly, and in good repair?
Equipment Condition	Is essential equipment in safe and effective operating condition?
Survey Posted	Are survey results readily accessible to residents?
Information Posted	Is information about Medicare, Medicaid, and contacting advocacy agencies posted?
Positioning	Is correct posture and comfortable positioning and assistance being provided to residents who need assistance?

Emergency	Are staff prepared for an emergency or disaster? Ask two staff and a charge nurse to describe what they do in emergencies.
Emergency Power	Is there emergency power?
Waste	Is waste contained in properly maintained cans, dumpsters, or compactors?

Source. Adapted from Form HCFA-803, July, 1995. Many statements are paraphrased.

APPENDIX H

Information to be Provided to a Surveyor Within One Hour or Twenty-Four Hours of the Entrance Conference

Within One Hour

1. List of key facility personnel and their locations.

2. A copy of the written information that is provided to residents regarding their rights.

3. Meal times and medication pass times.

4. List of admissions during the past month, and a list of the residents transferred or discharged during the past three months.

5. A copy of the facility's layout, indicating the location of nurses' stations, individual resident rooms, and common areas.

6. Activity calendar for last three months.

7. Menus of the food that will be served for the duration of the survey.

8. A copy of the facility admission contract.

9. A list of residents who have elected the hospice benefit and are currently receiving hospice care from an outside agency.

10. A list of residents who receive dialysis services.

11. The names of any residents age 55 and under.

12. The names of any residents who communicate with nonoral communication devices, sign language, or who speak a language other than the dominant language of the facility.

13. Evidence that the facility, on a routine basis, monitors accidents and other incidents, records these in the clinical or other record, and has a place to prevent and/or minimize further accidents and incidents.

Within Twenty-Four Hours

1. A completed Long-Term Care Facility Application for Medicare and Medicaid (HCFA-671); a Resident Census and Conditions of Residents (HCFA-672).

2. A list of Medicare residents who requested demand bills in the last six months (SNFs or dually participating SNF/Nfs only).

APPENDIX I
Scope and Severity Grid

	Isolated	Pattern	Widespread
Immediate Jeopardy to Resident Health or Safety	J	K	L
Actual Harm That Is Not Immediate Jeopardy	G	H	I
No Actual Harm with Potential for More Than Minimal Harm That Is Not Immediate Jeopardy	D	E	F
No Actual Harm with Potential for Minimal Harm	A	B	C

Source: HCFA, 1995, State Operations Manual, Transmittal 273.

Index

Page numbers followed by the letter "t" indicate a table; an "f" indicate a figure.

Order Your Own Copy of
This Important Book for Your Personal Library!

PSYCHOSOCIAL INTERVENTION IN LONG-TERM CARE
An Advanced Guide

_____ in hardbound at $49.95 (ISBN: 0-7890-0114-4)

_____ in softbound at $22.95 (ISBN: 0-7890-0189-6)

COST OF BOOKS _____

OUTSIDE USA/CANADA/
MEXICO: ADD 20% _____

POSTAGE & HANDLING _____
(US: $3.00 for first book & $1.25
for each additional book)
Outside US: $4.75 for first book
& $1.75 for each additional book)

SUBTOTAL _____

IN CANADA: ADD 7% GST _____

STATE TAX _____
(NY, OH & MN residents, please
add appropriate local sales tax)

FINAL TOTAL _____
(If paying in Canadian funds,
convert using the current
exchange rate. UNESCO
coupons welcome.)

☐ **BILL ME LATER:** ($5 service charge will be added)
(Bill-me option is good on US/Canada/Mexico orders only;
not good to jobbers, wholesalers, or subscription agencies.)

☐ Check here if billing address is different from
shipping address and attach purchase order and
billing address information.

Signature _____

☐ **PAYMENT ENCLOSED: $** _____

☐ **PLEASE CHARGE TO MY CREDIT CARD.**

☐ Visa   ☐ MasterCard   ☐ AmEx   ☐ Discover
☐ Diner's Club
Account # _____

Exp. Date _____

Signature _____

Prices in US dollars and subject to change without notice.

NAME _____

INSTITUTION _____

ADDRESS _____

CITY _____

STATE/ZIP _____

COUNTRY _____ COUNTY (NY residents only) _____

TEL _____ FAX _____

E-MAIL_____
May we use your e-mail address for confirmations and other types of information? ☐ Yes   ☐ No

Order From Your Local Bookstore or Directly From
The Haworth Press, Inc.
10 Alice Street, Binghamton, New York 13904-1580 • USA
TELEPHONE: 1-800-HAWORTH (1-800-429-6784) / Outside US/Canada: (607) 722-5857
FAX: 1-800-895-0582 / Outside US/Canada: (607) 772-6362
E-mail: getinfo@haworth.com
PLEASE PHOTOCOPY THIS FORM FOR YOUR PERSONAL USE.

BOF96